HOW DO I KNOW IF I HAVE FIBROMYALGIA?
Patients suffering from fibromyalgia experience a variety of painful and debilitating symptoms, including chronic fatigue, joint and muscle pain, chronic bladder and vaginal infections, depression, insomnia, and disorientation.

WHAT WERE THE TRADITIONAL REMEDIES?
Recognized as a disease by the World Health Organization in 1993, fibromyalgia has been treated in the past with medications to relieve symptoms, including antidepressants, analgesics, and narcotics. These remedies have not worked for everyone.

WHAT'S SO SPECIAL ABOUT GUAIFENESIN?
Guaifenesin is an inexpensive medication used in over-the-counter products for nasal congestion. But in his studies, Dr. St. Amand discovered that this drug, taken in the proper dosage, is the first effective treatment for reversing fibromyalgia—with no known side effects.

WHERE CAN I TURN FOR MORE INFORMATION—AND SUPPORT?
Dr. St. Amand is the country's foremost expert on this subject and is himself a past sufferer of the disease. Drawing on Dr. St. Amand's firsthand experience and filled with the latest research on the subject, this book also offers complete appendices that include Internet user groups and dozens of support organizations for people with fibromyalgia and for those using guaifenesin.

Please turn the page for more...

WHAT YOUR DOCTOR MAY *NOT* TELL YOU ABOUT

FIBROMYALGIA

THE REVOLUTIONARY TREATMENT THAT CAN REVERSE THE DISEASE

R. PAUL ST. AMAND, M.D., AND CLAUDIA CRAIG MAREK

WARNER BOOKS

A Time Warner Company

The information in this book can help you understand options for treatment, but is not intended to be a substitute for individual medical diagnosis and advice. You are advised to consult with your personal healthcare professional before implementing any program or therapy.

Copyright © 1999 R. Paul St. Amand, M.D., Claudia Craig Marek, M.A., and Mari Florence
All rights reserved.

Warner Books, Inc., 1271 Avenue of the Americas, New York, NY 10020
Visit our Web site at www.twbookmark.com

 A Time Warner Company

Printed in the United States of America
First Printing: December 1999
10 9 8 7 6 5 4

Library of Congress Cataloging-in-Publication Data

St. Amand, R. Paul.
    What your doctor may not tell you about fibromyalgia : the revolutionary
treatment that can reverse the disease / R. Paul St. Amand, and Claudia Craig Marek.
        p. cm.
    ISBN 0-446-67512-1
    1. Fibromyalgia. I. Marek, Claudia. II. Title.
RC927.3.S73 1999
616.7'4—dc21   99-24243
                                                                          CIP

Interior design by Charles Sutherland
Cover design by Rachel McClain

I dedicate this book to my wife, Janell, who endowed me with her support and love while sparing me time from the companionship I should have provided. I have bored her too frequently with my tales of fibromyalgia. I have required much understanding and acceptance: she gave me both.
R. Paul St. Amand, M.D.

To my husband Lou (who cooked me many dinners), and to my sons, Malcolm and Sean, for giving me the gift of time to write this book. To my sisters and parents for their love and support this busy year and all years. To all our patients and the Guai Group for their eloquent stories and insightful wisdom—I could not have done this without any of you.
Claudia Craig Marek

Contents

Foreword

In 1988, as an intern in the Bellevue Hospital Medical Clinic, I would see many patients who complained of generalized joint and muscle pain. Although these patients were frequently tender to touch, I could find no other abnormalities. I ordered many X rays and prescribed a lot of Tylenol and Motrin, and I eventually became frustrated with my inability to help these patients or even understand their illness. My colleagues were no better—even the supervising faculty had little understanding as to why the patients were experiencing chronic pain, and using terms like "total body pain."

Three years later, while studying for my medical boards, I came across the term "fibromyalgia." I immediately realized that many of the patients I had seen were suffering from the disease. I also realized that my lack of understanding of this illness had caused me to order many unnecessary tests, and prescribe medications that were of no help. There were a large number of doctors doing the same, and I knew that if I learned how to effectively treat fibromyalgia, I could make a difference in a lot of people's lives.

After finishing a fellowship in Rheumatology, I began my practice at the New York University Medical Center. I took an interest in treating fibromyalgia and soon began to see many patients with the illness. Although I had some success in treating my patients with a variety of muscle relaxants, sleep medications, anti-depressants, and painkillers, there was still a large number who remained ill. I was very frustrated by this, so I began to look for other ways to help these patients. Textbooks and journals offered no help. I then decided to search the Internet. Initially this increased my frustration—most sites offered either toxic medications, which appeared unlikely to help or were poorly disguised ads to sell medication. I then came across Dr. St. Amand's Web site. At first, I was skeptical that a medication as simple as guaifenesin could produce such impressive results. However, I was impressed with how well thought-out Dr. St. Amand's protocol was and was intrigued that I might be able to help my patients with this safe, inexpensive drug.

I immediately began treating a few of my patients with guaifenesin. At first due to the fact that I did not realize such a large number of products contained salicylates—substances that hinder guaifenesin from working—I had a low success rate. But then some of my patients began to get better, and the few who were able to completely avoid salicylates improved dramatically. A turning point in my treating fibromyalgia occurred when I finally spoke to Dr. St. Amand. I called him one day, and despite not knowing me, he immediately took my call. He explained how he began using guaifenesin, how to adjust the dosages, and what one needs to do so as to not prevent the medication from working—avoiding salicylates.

Armed with this new information I began to treat many more patients with guaifenesin. Remarkably, after an initial period of worsening, many of these patients began to improve. They not only experienced decreased pain, but also less fatigue and an increased level of concentration. The difficult part was teaching patients to properly avoid salicylates.

As you can imagine, I was being bombarded with questions about salicylates and which products contained them. But, Aileen Goldberg and Kristen Walters, two of my patients, came to my aid and formed a support group for fibromyalgia patients in New York City. There was now a resource for my patients' questions (in addition to Dr. St. Amand's Web site on the Internet). Besides information on salicylates and other treatments for fibromyalgia, the group also offered great support to other sufferers when they were in the midst of painful cycles.

My patients continue to improve with guaifenesin and every day I am grateful I have the opportunity to use this powerful medication. I am also grateful to have learned from such a dedicated man.

Finally, this past year I had the opportunity to meet Dr. St. Amand. It was an honor to speak with such a compassionate and caring man, one who has devoted his life to helping patients with fibromyalgia. I had a chance to learn his mapping techniques and to "fine tune" my use of guaifenesin.

While many of the other medications I use may improve the pain and fatigue of fibromyalgia, guaifenesin offers patients the possibility to actually reverse the illness. This book should be the beginning of the road to health for many with fibromyalgia.

Bruce M. Solitar, M.D.
Clinical Assistant Professor of Medicine
Division of Rheumatology
New York University Medical Center

Preface

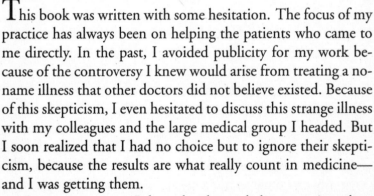

This book was written with some hesitation. The focus of my practice has always been on helping the patients who came to me directly. In the past, I avoided publicity for my work because of the controversy I knew would arise from treating a no-name illness that other doctors did not believe existed. Because of this skepticism, I even hesitated to discuss this strange illness with my colleagues and the large medical group I headed. But I soon realized that I had no choice but to ignore their skepticism, because the results are what really count in medicine—and I was getting them.

I was on my own. I drew sketches to help my patients better understand their disease and the course of treatment I recommended. However, my "fibrofogged" patients needed something written to review and to bring home to their families. It became necessary to write descriptive patient papers. These were copied and circulated among many fibromyalgics who were not my patients, as well as their friends, their cousins, and their neighbors. In my wildest dreams I could not have anticipated the number of patients these papers would bring to my office from all over the United States and eventually from around the world.

When the name "fibromyalgia" was coined about seventeen years ago, I gratefully adopted this nomenclature—misnomer though it was! Finally, a "real" name was given to this old disease and helped it to gain acceptance from some members of the medical community. This led to my coming out of the closet, since now the disease "officially" existed. Though my approach was unconventional and not in accordance with the party line, I was increasingly asked to speak and write about my experiences with fibromyalgia and its associated conditions, the most prevalent of these being hypoglycemia (or low blood sugar), a common accompaniment to fibromyalgia.

As I studied and learned more about the nameless disease we now call fibromyalgia, I realized that I also had it. Later, I was able to identify the condition as one of my father's legacies. It was he who carried the gene and unwittingly passed it on to my two sisters and me. Over the span of a few years, I realized that, one by one, each of my three daughters were developing the same symptoms as they grew older. Illnesses take on special significance when they strike near to home. My family's traits obviously drove me to hone my skills a bit more sharply.

Over the years we used five medications before recently discovering the most effective and safest one. After my success with the earliest drug, I began to wonder why it worked. This "why?" led to possibilities and then to theories, which I occasionally changed and modified, and will continue to do so. A theory is merely a supposition based on as much fact as can be garnered. Errors in our theory would not alter the success of our treatment. My working hypothesis has enhanced my pleasure of poring over esoteric papers that provide monthly, new, and exciting data on cellular physiology. Perhaps a simpler statement is: *What works, works.* In fact, the heart of my approach is so basic that it can be stated in a simple quartet of phrases:

1. There is an inherited disease known as the fibromyalgia syndrome (FMS)—a name that is actually a misnomer.

2. There exists an effective, safe treatment using a very old medication, guaifenesin.

3. The inability to form adequate energy in affected tissues explains the entire spectrum of the illness.

4. Hypoglycemia, or low blood sugar, is a frequent co-condition.

This book was written from elements of both despair and dedication. Despair has come with my age and my concern about the dissemination of my more than forty years of experience treating fibromyalgia. Dedication translates into the urgent need to get information to the countless patients who must take responsibility for the success of their own treatment. Patients rely on their physicians to diagnose their illnesses and ease their symptoms. We urge them to find one who will work with them and follow this protocol using what I see as a miracle drug, guaifenesin. At the same time, it is unrealistic for patients to expect these doctors to help them without helping themselves—this means following the program outlined in this book very carefully.

I understand there will be those who will claim that we

wrote this book only for its commercial value. Others, more academic in their criticism, will point to the fact that our treatment protocol using guaifenesin has not been subjected to a successful, double-blind study. More technically skilled critics will wonder how we can assume so much by delving into the realm of deep-seated biochemistry using so little evidence. Some of these skeptics will undoubtedly feel that our use of a particularly simple medication to reverse a particularly complex illness is simplistic.

It is proper for me to respond to each criticism in turn. First, I do trust this venture will be profitable. I see no harm in the good, old-fashioned, enterprising approach. Second, an attempt to show the success of our treatment with a double-blind study was carried out at the University of Oregon, but it failed due to some errors—errors we now know how to fix. As a consultant on this study I share the blame. The first error came from my own ignorance regarding certain compounds that blocked the effectiveness of the guaifenesin that we were testing. The second error was the failure to keep hypo-glycemics out of the study. Yet I hasten to assure the generous Scott family, who funded this project, that the knowledge we gained has helped us immensely although, unfortunately, we still lack the gold standard of a successful study. But we will try to change that in the near future.

Lastly, I would also like to address the concerns of the chemically sophisticated minority. Please be aware that the chemistry I describe is up to date only as of this writing. We believe that future developments in biochemistry will show our theory is reasonably correct. If we are right, some of the mysteries surrounding fibromyalgia will soon be unveiled.

I was inspired to write this book for the millions of untreated patients, many of whom suffer terribly and are desperate for knowledge. We try to answer the hundreds of letters and e-mail that pour into our office, but we must also leave time to see our own patients and answer many phone calls. Every day we hear sad and complex stories. I can also recall a myriad of faces, wounded psyches, destroyed relationships, and tragic complaints from my four decades in private practice. I remember especially the times we failed. But all solutions come about through a process of trial and error.

Thankfully our success rate has improved as we have learned from our patient-teachers. Their perceptions of seemingly insignificant nuances and their eagerness to share their experiences have proved invaluable to us all. I dedicate this book to the patients who stood by us and taught us during our trial-and-error phase. They were and are the flesh and blood of my concepts of fibromyalgia and "fibroglycemia." They have helped me provide you with the lifesaving program outlined in this book. I thank them, and I know you will too.

—R. Paul St. Amand, M.D.

Acknowledgments

I bow to my nurse and coauthor, Claudia Marek, who has filled this book with her intelligent perceptions. She has provided years of inspiration, not only for me, but also for all of our patients, with her caring and deep knowledge of these illnesses. I am in awe of both of my two other writing colleagues, Mari Florence and Skye Van Raalte-Herzog, who labored mightily to "keep things simple" in the hopes of softening my medical jargon to the realm of the understandable. Our editor Diana Baroni, who labored with skill and enthusiasm, is also owed a heartfelt thanks. There is not enough room to express gratitude to all of our friends and families, especially Lou, Malcolm, and Sean, who patiently added their art and observations while they allowed us to steal monumental time from our relationships. Lastly, another stands out as a mighty contributor: my secretary, Gloria Martinez, who has efficiently and uncomplainingly assumed many mundane duties that freed nurse and doctor to pursue this endeavor.

WHAT YOUR DOCTOR MAY *NOT* TELL YOU ABOUT

FIBROMYALGIA

Part I

THE PLAN FOR CONQUERING FIBROMYALGIA

The first part of this book is an invitation. We will tell you about fibromyalgia, and about ourselves, and what this book has to offer you. We will explain what we do and why we do it, so that you can decide for yourself if you're a candidate for our protocol. Even if you think you might not be, this book has lots of useful information about fibromyalgia itself. We have a whole chapter about the medication we use, and another about the things you need to know before you start using it. There's a chapter on hypoglycemia, or low blood sugar, because so many fibromyalgics have this problem. It will help you decide if you need to be on the diet and then explains what the diet is. The last chapter is a concise step-by-step explanation of the protocol, one that you can refer back to when you have questions.

Chapter 1

An Invitation to Join Us and Find Your Way Back to Health

Having fibromyalgia means many things change, and a lot of them are invisible. Unlike having cancer or being hurt in an accident, most people do not understand even a little about (this illness) and its effects, and of those that think they know, many are actually misinformed.

—J. M., Texas

It can start off quite subtly: a bit of muscle pain, along with some generalized aches and stiffness. Then there are periods when concentration is impossible, a day or two of overwhelming fatigue, and maybe a little dizziness, cramps, and diarrhea. Symptoms come and go at first, and it's easy to chalk them up to a mild case of flu that never quite localizes, to overexertion and too much stress in your life.

Then, one day, you realize it hasn't gone away—it never goes away anymore. One part or another of your body always hurts. You feel stressed and irritable all of the time. You wake up tired every morning. In short, you haven't felt "right" in a long time. The symptoms begin to worsen, and you notice new ones. Perhaps depression, numbness and tingling of the hands, leg cramps, stiffness, headaches, or bladder infections. Often you can no longer sleep through the night. Sometimes it's pain that keeps you awake; sometimes you don't know what it is that keeps you from falling asleep. When you do sleep, you wake up tired and unrefreshed. You crave sugar or other carbohydrates, and if you give in to this craving, you tend to gain weight and feel even worse. Then, before you know it, bad days outweigh the good ones, and eventually there are no good days, just ones that range from bad to worse.

> It feels like coming down with the flu, yet it never manifests fully. It's like being fluish, achy and tired, and embarrassed and discouraged about it because you don't know why or what you can do to make it better or what you did to make it worse. Everyone gives advice but they don't have a clue as to what it's really like. Having people tell you to eat differently and exercise more and not focus on your health makes you just want to isolate yourself because you've already experimented with every possible food plan, supplement, and idea.
>
> —*Miki K., Hawaii*

You become increasingly immobile. Gradually and without realizing it at first, you stop making plans because you never know how you will feel, and you become mostly housebound or bedridden. The simple task of going to the supermarket can be an impossible chore. By now you have visited doctors of various specialties in the hope that one of them will be able to tell you what's wrong and set things right. When the pain is bad, you seek out chiropractors and massage therapists, and maybe you try acupuncture and alternative treatments like herbs or homeopathy. You have had many diagnostic tests run, costing hundreds, perhaps even thousands of dollars. Your friends have offered you a lot of advice about vitamins and nutritional supplements that have helped them or someone they know. But you are already taking a regimen of vitamins, minerals, and enzymes, and you do not feel much better. You may have heard the word "fibromyalgia," and maybe you know whether or not you have it. No one has told you how to treat your disease, although they have many ideas about how to ease your symptoms.

Your life has entered a downward spiral of pain, depression, and fatigue. You have a great deal of guilt about not being the person you used to be. Unless you are blessed with an exceptional companion, your personal relationships have suffered or completely fallen apart. You worry about your ability to care for your children. You may even contemplate suicide.

> It feels like everyone around me is normal and happy and having a good time and I'm so different. I want to have a few normal days. I don't fit in anywhere because no one understands. People laugh and say "You look fine" but I'm dying inside and I can't explain it to them. I'm so tired of pretending I'm okay when I want to scream. I have kept a positive attitude for so long but it's exhausting and I just can't do it anymore. I wish I could just go away somewhere and hide.
>
> —*Susie*

This is an oversimplified picture of what it's like to have fibromyalgia. Those of you who have it know that it is far more involved than this. I know what you're going through. I am intimately familiar with the personal struggles that each and every one of you has experienced with this illness either as sufferers or as their supporters. I have lived with your pain, your fatigue, and your despair.

I have spent my entire medical career treating patients with symptoms such as these and more. Headaches, jaw and facial pain, abdominal discomfort, dizziness, memory lapses, vulvar and bladder pain, itching and rashes, all plague fibromyalgics. Until recently, doctors told patients like you that your illness was due to "nerves." And, to underscore this diagnosis, patients were reminded that the pages and pages of tests run on them had shown "nothing wrong."

Fibromyalgia is prevalent in all ethnic groups in all parts of the world. In North America, it is estimated that about five percent of the adult population suffers from this disease, although I believe the actual rate is higher. Conservatively then, some twenty million Americans suffer from fibromyalgia and its related disorders—most are women, with the ratio of women to men at about five to one. There is some evidence, mostly anecdotal, that this statistic may be skewed due to the fact that men are often either misdiagnosed or less likely to visit a doctor. Rheumatologists say fibromyalgia is the most common disorder they see.[1]

Another twenty-five million people suffer from chronic fatigue syndrome, which I (and most other physicians) believe is the same disease. I have good reasons to conclude through my work that today's fibromyalgia is the prelude to tomorrow's osteoarthritis that afflicts another thirty-five million people. Adding these numbers would suggest that one third of our population will suffer with some of the symptoms of fibromyalgia at some point in their lives. And this does not include those who have been diagnosed with other "syndromes," such as myofascial pain, chronic candidiasis, vulvar pain, irritable bowel and irritable bladder, and so on—who in all probability have fibromyalgia as well.

> My rheumatologist told me I was too old to have FMS. At that time I was fifty-four, never mind the fact I had had symptoms most of my life. The disease had become "full blown" when I was about fifty-one. . . . After another year of suffering, I diagnosed myself via the Net. My DO (Doctor of Osteopathy) sent me back to the same rheumatologist because he is the only board-certified one in our area. At that time he told me I was too old to have FMS but even if I did there was nothing that could be done. . . . I have since been diagnosed with FMS by three other doctors, all of whom have told me the only thing they could do was treat my symptoms. I was as good as I would ever be and would get much worse.
>
> —*Betty, Texas*

"Rheumatism with painful hard places" which can be felt in various locations on the body is considered the first description of fibromyalgia in modern medical texts, by a doctor named Froriep in 1843. Sir William Gowers of University College Hospital in London, who began by studying his own lumbago, initially dubbed this disease "fibrositis" in 1904.[2] Dr. Gowers observed that his patients were also exhausted and that the disease was "so painful it would make a strong man cry out." He tried everything he could think of in an attempt to relieve this pain, including injecting cocaine into the tender points (it didn't work very well) and having patients take a newly discovered drug called aspirin that, he observed, didn't work very well either.[3] "Fibromyalgia," a Greek word meaning pain in the muscles, has now all but erased fibrositis and rheumatism as the name of this disease.

On New Year's Day 1993, fibromyalgia was officially declared a syndrome by the World Health Organization (WHO) in the Copenhagen Declaration. It was declared the most common cause of widespread chronic muscle pain. As a new entry in the ICD code (International Statistical Classification of Diseases and Related Health Problems) it became an official diagnosis that, among other things, a doctor could use to bill insurance companies and to label a patient disabled. The WHO decided to incorporate into the definition of the disease the American College of Rheumatology's 1990 definition penned by Drs. Muhammed Yunus, Hugh Smythe, and Frederick Wolfe.[4] This had carefully detailed the location of eighteen tender points symmetrically located around the human body. The presence of at least eleven out of eighteen of these was considered the gold standard for diagnosis, along with muscle pain.

But the World Health Organization went a little farther. The Copenhagen Declaration added: "Fibromyalgia is part of a wider syndrome encompassing headaches, irritable bladder, dysmenorrhea, cold sensitivity, Reynaud's phenomenon, restless legs, atypical patterns of numbness and tingling, exercise intolerance, and complaints of weakness." It also recognized that patients are often depressed.[5]

Today, thousands of medical articles later, fibromyalgia is almost universally recognized as a distinct illness. Sadly, there remain a few doctors who still try to tell patients it is simply a catchall name for a collection of symptoms shared by a group of neurotic women, but luckily they are increasingly rare. Despite so many articles and so much speculation, much of fibromyalgia remains poorly understood. It is a complex and chronic disease that causes widespread pain and profound fatigue—accompanied by a range of symptoms that make simple, everyday tasks daunting, difficult, and sometimes even impossible.

> Once upon a time, a lifetime ago, I was a gymnast, played in tennis leagues, golfed, played on a softball team, and panned for gold in the Colorado mountains. . . . Now I am lucky if I can walk to my mailbox—usually I have to drive. If I can make the stairs, I go down to check on the laundry situation, or go upstairs to see if the dust has carried away the entire floor.
> —*Gloria*

Symptoms affect widely disparate parts of the body. Doctors don't always realize that tenderness in the neck area, frequent bladder infections, and brittle nails, for example, are symptoms of the same illness. Patients, often young women, look "well" and many have learned to put up a façade in the workplace or with friends. A growing number of people have now heard of fibromyalgia and know someone who has it. Lists are available that detail the multiple symptoms of the disease, but it remains a phantom illness that has few concrete findings to the casual examiner. It still lacks a laboratory test to confirm its existence, and no scans or X rays can detect it. For these reasons, fibromyalgia is often described as an "invisible disability."

Yet a well-conducted history will unveil the chronology of the cyclic symptoms that point to a diagnosis. This is easily confirmed by the many abnormalities in muscles, tendons, and ligaments revealed by a detailed examination. Some doctors enjoy semantics and argue whether this is a syndrome or a true disease. "Disease" is exactly that: *lack of ease,* and fibromyalgics are certainly qualified to wear that name. Symptoms and findings that regularly appear together in a number of patients are grouped as a "syndrome." Congratulations! Fibromyalgia is that, too.

The painful areas of tenderness are often superimposed at the sites of previous injuries or surgery, so some believe that it is caused by trauma. We believe that there are good scientific reasons why this should be, but we also believe the disease-syndrome is inherited. Since eighty-five percent of fibromyalgia patients are women, at least one gene is undoubtedly on the X chromosome. But there must be more than one gene involved, since we have seen the illness begin as early as the age of four and as late as the age of seventy-four. That spread would be impossible to explain with only one defective gene.

> There is no doubt in my mind that there is a genetic predisposition to FMS. My eighty-six-year-old father has had it since my teen years. My mother recently told me when I asked about his leg pain that the doctor said years ago that there were lumps in his legs.
> —*M. Bush, Alabama*

Although fibromyalgia is not a terminal illness, it is a demoralizing and debilitating one. The symptoms can be unbearable—so unbearable that the so-called "Suicide Doctor,"

Dr. Kevorkian, has helped several fibromyalgia patients end their suffering. In 1997, one of these fibromyalgics was forty-year-old Janis Murphy. After her death, her father spoke out about his daughter's condition. "Over the years, I've seen my daughter experience intractable and unrelenting pain." He hated losing his only child, but "there are things in this world worse than death."

The currently accepted method for helping fibromyalgics is to recommend exercise (knowing the patient can't do it) and to employ a war chest full of chemical Band-Aids used simply to palliate the lengthening litany of symptoms. Medical professionals unwittingly promote increasing disability when they prescribe ever-stronger medications that, sooner or later, deplete energy even further and deepen the mental haze. Along with the failure of exercise programs, massage, and physiotherapy, patients accept their lot and become victims of their disease.

To make bad matters even worse, long-term disability insurance companies have now entered the fibromyalgia fray and help to confound progress. It is to their advantage to insist that the disease and all of its variations stem from psychiatric disorders. They often have no difficulty in finding a psychiatrist who will agree. Since the vast majority of insurance policies do not cover mental disability beyond a specified time, there is a great deal of money at stake. Fibromyalgia cases have reached near epidemic proportions in the form of U.S. Social Security disability claims, workers' compensations, and accident litigation. As many as twenty-five percent of American fibromyalgia patients have received some form of disability or injury compensation.[6] We are first to agree that the country can ill afford to swell these ranks. But we cannot turn our back on very real suffering, either.

Although there is no consensus as to the source of the disease, I postulate throughout this book, hopefully in simple enough terms, that it is caused by an abnormality in phosphate excretion. As I have already suggested, this inherited problem appears to me to be due to a genetic defect. Retention of phosphates eventually interferes with energy formation in affected cells. Patients describe their lack of energy, and cellular metabolism confirms it. If there is insufficient energy, "nothing works right"—the very complaint of the fibromyalgic. Pick a cell, any cell, from a system that bothers you, strip it of its energy, and you won't find it hard to explain why the brain, muscles, tendons, ligaments, intestine, urinary tract, and skin have joined in an act of biochemical vandalism.

Fibromyalgia is a nearly total, systemwide illness in most patients. The seemingly unconnected shifts in complaints confuses physicians, who respond by referring patients to another doctor who knows more about the "new" symptom. In the process, patients often receive a sort of medical education as they move from specialist to specialist.

Physicians are well intentioned, dedicated, and skillfully trained in trying to find ways to help their patients. I assure you that they are frequently frustrated and stymied by the difficulties fibromyalgia presents. And then, the consensus among most of my colleagues is that fibromyalgia is incurable. This makes it acceptable to relieve symptoms by reliance on medications such as NSAIDs (nonsteroidal anti-inflammatory drugs), narcotics, analgesics, and mood-altering drugs. This polypharmacy often complicates the patient's condition by further depressing the central nervous system, causing more fatigue and mental confusion. The result is that patients are even less able to control their lives than they were before treatment.

In my years as an internist and endocrinologist, I have devoted much of my career to the diagnosis and treatment of this disease. I have found that there is an effective, safe treatment for fibromyalgia, and I have used it myself. Fibromyalgia entered my own life when I was in the service in 1945. I was hospitalized with the diagnosis of "possible rheumatic fever." All my tests were normal, though, and after six weeks my swollen muscles and joints cleared. Cycles of these symptoms were sporadic for years after that, until I was in my early thirties and they returned in earnest. Since I had no idea what was bothering me and I knew of no disease that would cause such ridiculous symptoms, I assumed I was not geared for the tribulations of having a private medical practice. I tried to pace myself and relax as best I could. It was only after I began treating patients with the disease that was later to be called fibromyalgia that I realized that I shared their misery, and began to treat myself.

Over the years I have explored the many facets of this illness mainly through observation and the compilation of data from my patient-teachers. They willingly joined me in our trial-and-error approach that lacked any other scientific credentials. It has taken many years for me to reasonably grasp the full extent of this illness and to comprehend just how insidious it can be.

I have used several different drugs to treat fibromyalgia. In the past I used exclusively gout medications and, though effective, each had certain side effects which left in limbo a small group of patients who could not tolerate them. In 1992, the continuing search led me to guaifenesin, a widely available medication. It has no known side effects, is well tolerated, and has no remaining patent and is therefore inexpensive.

I have used guaifenesin to develop a treatment protocol that addresses the actual disturbance caused by our defective genes, not merely its symptoms. This book is the culmination of nearly four decades of research. I have treated thousands of patients who have traveled from all over the world seeking relief from this enervating disease. With treatment, the symptoms and pain reverse and disappear completely in most patients. Other patients resume normal lives with minimal residual problems. This is not to say that recovery occurs immediately. Not only is it necessary to find the effective dosage of guaifenesin, there are also other crucial factors that influence the outcome of my treatment.

Briefly, in order for guaifenesin to work, it must have unrestricted access to receptors in the kidneys, the little garages where the medication must park if it is going to work. Many ingredients in the products we use every day—lipsticks, muscle balms, nutritional and herbal supplements, cosmetics, toothpastes, and sunscreens—are chemicals known as "salicylates." These totally block the guaifenesin's access to the renal receptors where it works. When this access is blocked, none of the drugs we use are of any benefit whatsoever. Thus salicylates must be carefully avoided.

It also must be understood that approximately forty percent of female fibromyalgics have hypoglycemia, or low blood sugar, and symptoms overlap those of fibromyalgia. To be successful, treatment must address both conditions simultaneously. If this connection is overlooked and the patient fails to make the necessary dietary adjustments, the symptoms of hypoglycemia remain.

For these reasons, my protocol, as laid out in this book, should be followed very carefully in order to achieve positive results. Despite the need to watch carefully for blockers, there is no treatment currently available that is as safe or has enjoyed such a high level of success.

In succeeding chapters of this book, I will discuss all of the important factors a patient must address to successfully treat fibromyalgia, as well as share my knowledge of the disease itself. Guaifenesin is so safe that it is an ingredient in many over-the-counter cold and allergy medicines. It should be taken daily and in an appropriate dosage. Patients of any age can follow the protocol, which is designed to reverse fibromyalgia in less time than it took to develop. This book will also discuss some coping strategies. There is no question that the unrelenting nature of the disease, the cognitive losses, the fatigue, and the pains are certainly reason enough to induce depression and even suicidal thoughts. To cope with this horrible disease, patients do need more than a pill and the instructions about how to take it.

The guaifenesin approach to fibromyalgia is not well known or currently widely accepted. Since we have been unable to publish in medical journals, its fame derives entirely from grassroots support and the militancy of the patients it has helped. The list of physicians all over the country who use and support our protocol has grown to about two hundred. Many more are allowing patients to use the drug, as we constantly learn from our e-mail postings and letters from all over the world. We have spoken to hundreds of doctors who have called our office. Many more have written for information. My coauthor and I have spoken to groups in many parts of the country and have delivered our message about the success of guaifenesin to anyone who will listen. This book is, to us, merely a means to help many more people than we could ever hope to do in person. There is no doubt whatsoever that guaifenesin is highly effective as long as users exercise care in following our instructions.

> To the guai army: this treatment will go forth into the world as long as we keep standing our ground. Guai works! Each time a doctor becomes convinced of the effectiveness of guaifenesin, he will spread the word to his other patients and their families. We began as a small voice crying in the night. Each day we are getting louder through the strength of our numbers. Our family grows and the world is a better place.
>
> —*Kathy Shuller, Florida*

We also know that each patient must take charge of his or her own illness. Physicians will continue having difficulty coping with the many hidden sources of salicylates. It is hardly their job to walk around cosmetic counters reading labels with a magnifying glass as we have done. That task will continue to be the patient's problem. It is also the patient's responsibility to adhere to the hypoglycemia diet, if that is necessary. Cheating on the diet will harm not only you, but also affects the assessment of the doctor who is watching you for positive results—and all the other patients who rely on his or her knowledge.

The fact that you are reading this book says a lot. You are still motivated to try. You have already overpaid your dues, and we aim to help you restore your health.

I began noticeable symptoms of fibromyalgia in July 1990. . . . My symptoms began as burning on the bottoms of my feet and then within months progressed to my ankles, legs, hips, and lower back. I began to get such symptoms as headaches, muscle spasms, fatigue, and others. After seeing about twenty different doctors, no help was found, and it was said that the pain was all in my head. I was harassed into leaving my job because I had not been coming to work off and on for a year and a half. . . . Then, in July of 1993 . . . I began taking guaifenesin. . . . In the first week or two, I had had some terribly painful days. But gradually they got less and less painful and I began seeing a good day here and there. My "good" days became more and more frequent. I am currently about ninety-percent improved from using the guaifenesin treatment for four years.

—*Nancy Medeiros, Escondido, CA*

I invite all fibromyalgia sufferers to embark upon a journey to improved health. Let us be your tour directors. We are passionate about providing you with the information you need to regain your vitality. Realize up front that this journey is not for the faint of heart. For most of you, the road back to good health will seem long, with days of pain and discomfort. In the beginning, this may be more severe than what you have suffered to date.

Guaifenesin treatment flushes metabolic debris out of the body, and while this occurs, your pain will probably increase. Gradually you will notice that the days of pain and fatigue diminish, and good hours will eventually be followed by great days. You will bounce back again with energy after an illness, injury, or hard work, as you once did. You will be delighted that you can participate in activities with a strength that has eluded you for years. By following my treatment regimen to the letter, along with your doctor's advice, this is within your reach, and you can once again live life to its fullest. My ultimate goal is to ease the suffering and pain associated with this illness and, through this book, I hope to reach as many of you as possible with a viable and effective treatment solution. The best definition of happiness I have ever heard was: "Happiness is freedom from pain." Wipe out mental anguish as well as physical pain, and life is a joy.

🐚

Chapter 2

The Fibromyalgia Syndrome:
An Overview of Symptoms and Causes

These are the things I would like you to understand about me. Please understand that being sick doesn't mean I'm not a human being. I spend most of my day in considerable pain and exhaustion. Please understand the difference between happy and healthy. If you're talking to me and I sound happy, it means I'm happy. It doesn't mean that I'm not in a lot of pain, or extremely tired, or that I'm getting better, or any of those things.

Please understand that FMS is variable. One day I am able to walk to the park and back, the next day I'll have trouble getting to the kitchen. Please understand that "getting out and doing things" does not make me feel better, and can often make me feel seriously worse. Telling me that I need a treadmill, or that I just need to lose or gain weight, use an exercise machine, join a gym, go to exercise classes may frustrate me to tears and is not correct. If I was capable of doing these things, I would. I am not depressed, though I suffer from depression (wouldn't you if you were hurting and exhausted for years on end?). FM is not created by depression.

— *Based on an open letter by Bek Oberin*

🐚 WHAT IS FIBROMYALGIA?

What is fibromyalgia? This is the question for which everyone wants an answer. My nurse and coauthor, Claudia, asked her son, Malcolm Potter, that question when he was about ten years old. His response was: "It feels like all my muscles want to throw up!" This seems like a bright and descriptive answer. Another good one is: "The irritable everything syndrome," coined by Dr. Hugh Smythe of Canada.[7]

Fibromyalgia is different from other illnesses. Describing thyroid diseases, diabetes, or rheumatoid arthritis, for example, I can easily outline their distinguishing characteristics. Most conditions have a single set or series of lab tests that help confirm their diagnosis. This is not so with fibromyalgia because it does not affect one particular type of cell or part of the body. Instead, it is manifested by a myriad of what appear to be unrelated symptoms in an almost endless number of combinations. At first glance, the only thing these complaints seem to have in common is that they are in the same body. Because of their variety, these symptoms can't be neatly categorized into one or another of the usual medical specialty areas in which physicians operate. This may also contribute to fibromyalgia's elusiveness.

We can say that fibromyalgia is unique because it affects so many parts of the body and each patient's prime complaints are different. For this reason, patients seek help from whatever specialist appears best suited to handle their most pressing problem. Specialists, by definition, work in a more limited sphere, and so can easily get trapped into focusing only on the symptoms within their field. When they do not expand their perspective to view the entire patient presentation, they end up treating symptoms as if they were the entire entity. This is the reason why irritable bowel syndrome, interstitial cystitis, vulvar pain syndrome, chronic fatigue syndrome, chronic candidiasis, myofascial pain syndrome, and so on are treated separately, when they are not a disease, but names for a complex of symptoms. We have come to see each of them as a facet of fibromyalgia. So it is that physicians who are accustomed to performing complete patient evaluations, such as family practice specialists, internists, and rheumatologists, are the most adept in deciphering the nuances of fibromyalgia by connecting the head bone to the toe bone.

To illustrate how difficult this task can be, let us first look at these symptoms without discussing how they may be connected. This is the environment in which I practiced for much of my career. I spoke to patients who had numerous complaints, had visited many doctors, taken many medications, but still were not well, and had become progressively more frustrated. Family and friends had finally attributed their symptoms to neurosis or hypochondriasis. Their family doctor examined and tested them, often in detail, and ultimately supported the case for "nothing wrong but bad nerves." The connecting thread, common among patients, was the litany of complaints and the length of the list. The title of their recitation might have been "I haven't felt like myself in years." Patients found it difficult to pinpoint exactly when the symptoms began, let alone the order they came in: migraines, fatigue, muscle aches, dizziness, nasal congestion, gas, numbness, bladder infections, and the list goes on.

> Some mornings I would wake up and feel so lethargic it was all I could do to make it to work. For several years, I'd attributed my muscle pain to the few fender benders that I'd been in. I'd thought the migraine headaches were hereditary. And I would tell myself I'd caught a "bug" when the dizziness and fatigue became a problem. The strange thing was, the symptoms

seemed to get worse as time went on, not better, despite the treatment I'd received from traditional MDs, chiropractors, holistic practitioners, acupuncturists, masseuses, and herbalists.

About a year ago, I was so frustrated I rattled off all my recurring symptoms to my [previous] doctor and demanded, "I've been here before with these problems. What's wrong with me?" To which she replied with annoying frankness, "I don't know."

—*Michelle Fisher, Torrance, CA*

Other patients' histories centered on different types of complaints, but years of pain and misery always seemed to be the constant factor.

Like most disorders, the impact of fibromyalgia differs from patient to patient. Some patients are able to lead relatively normal lives. Others become homebound, and some become completely debilitated. Many fibromyalgics may feel fine until some traumatic event occurs, such as a car accident or an emotional setback. Then they begin to notice symptoms that never go away. Some fibromyalgics live with their symptoms for years, until finally they succumb to excruciating pain.

In addition to the physical complaints, many patients also have difficulties with memory and concentration—cognitive difficulties, nicknamed "fibrofog." These symptoms take as much of a toll on the patient as do the physical disturbances. They raise the fear of premature and serious brain deterioration. One can appreciate the severity of the neurological component of fibromyalgia with this account of the confusion and disorientation experienced by one sufferer:

I sit at a computer at work with a headset on, answering calls from people about computers of all types. . . . I have to solve their problems, at the same time "teach" them. Many times I have found myself not knowing who I am talking to (man or woman?) and what we were talking about. It is like just waking up from a dream. So I have to keep notes of what I'm doing on my calls, or just plain ask the person to repeat what they just said. This will eventually cost me my job . . . I don't know what my future holds. I've gotten in my car and forgotten how to turn the lights on, or where the windshield wipers are. Sometimes I can laugh about it, later. But it's getting more frequent and I'm not laughing anymore.

—*Cyndi S., Hot Springs, AR*

In my early days in practice, I knew of no disease that would include all of the weird symptoms expressed to me by my patients. From the sheer number of them who presented the same complaints, I became progressively more certain that some new disease had to exist. The frequent cycling from good to bad days in the early phases of the illness made it very unlikely that I was dealing with a neurosis. I noticed with all these patients that the tensions and stress levels of home life or working conditions made little difference as to when sick days would appear. Neurotics are always neurotic and they don't suddenly experience great days out of nowhere. The fact that my patients were inexplicably better at times made me start paying attention and tabulating symptoms.

Almost all of these patients complained of varying levels of physical pain in all parts of their bodies. This seemed tangible and thus a good place to start. I began to feel for abnormalities in painful areas. Not only did I find them, but I discovered that when patients were in pain, their other symptoms were worse too. Soon it became obvious that the entire cascade of symptoms were related and were connected to the physical changes I was learning to palpate. I started grouping symptoms into various systems and tried to link them into one disease with a single cause. When one grasps how many distinct parts of the body are affected, it is quite easy to understand how elusive the diagnosis of fibromyalgia can be for both patient and physician.

The Symptoms of Fibromyalgia

By and large, fibromyalgia symptoms can be grouped into the following categories: cerebral, musculoskeletal, dermal, gastrointestinal, and genitourinary. There are a few other, isolated problems that do not fit easily into any classification. Now let's look at each area that is affected and the tableau of symptoms a fibromyalgic may experience. Each of these groups merits a chapter later in this book to help you better understand your body and your complaints, and how guaifenesin will help them. But for now, let's just take a general overview.

Cerebral—Fatigue, irritability, nervousness, depression, impaired memory and concentration (this is also known as "fibrofog"), apathy, frequent awakening during the night, nonrestorative sleep, blurring of vision, dizziness, and headaches (often called migraines when they are sufficiently intense).

Musculoskeletal—Widespread, aching pain and stiffness in muscles, tendons and ligaments, which are often worse upon awakening. Pains can assume any form and intensity, such as throbbing, burning, stabbing, stinging, grabbing, or any combination of these. Numbness of the extremities or face and tingling anywhere are usually from contracted structures pressing on nearby nerves. Temporomandibular joint pain, possibly with difficult chewing, and excruciating facial and head pain originating in the neck are likewise common complaints. Muscles can often be seen twitching, and the restless leg syndrome can make it impossible to find a comfortable spot. Patients also complain of feelings like electrical impulses in their muscles, and a feeling of general weakness.

Dermal—Crawling feelings, itching, rashes (many varieties), burning, and sometimes swollen and hot-itching palms and soles of feet. Patients can have patches of pimples, and perspiration is both pungent and irritates the skin.

Gastrointestinal—(fibrogut) irritable bowel syndrome that includes gas, pain, bloating, constipation alternating with diarrhea, and sometimes, nausea or hyperacidity.

Genitourinary—Vulvodynia, which includes vulvitis (raw, irritated, burning vaginal lips) and vulvar pain, vaginal spasms or cramps, burning discharge, increased menstrual and uterine cramps, painful intercourse (dyspareunia), repeated bladder infections, pungent, concentrated urine, and chronic interstitial cystitis.

Miscellaneous—Excessive nasal congestion and mucus, brittle nails, inferior hair quality and dryness, dry, scalded, or metallic mouth sensations, eye irritation or blurring with a discharge or burning tears, and transient ringing in the ears or other sounds. Dizziness and true vertigo arise in the middle ear. Patients often complain of increased sensitivity to sounds, bright light, smells, and certain chemicals.

TENDER POINTS

Ever since the 1840s, when "painful hard places" were described in patients with rheumatism, both doctors and patients have been fascinated by them. These painful areas are now referred to as "tender points" (sometimes you'll hear them called trigger points, although this term is usually reserved for myofascial pain). The official (American Academy of Rheumatology) diagnostic criteria for fibromyalgia is based on the ability of the examiner to find eleven out of eighteen places in predetermined areas that are painful when pressed upon. These spots have been mapped, poked, prodded, biopsied, injected, and scanned. They are commonly assessed with a special contraption called a dolorimeter, a spring-loaded device designed to provide a measurement for the point at which the patient cries out or flinches.

When questioned, most patients describe tender areas throughout their bodies, located on or near muscles, tendons, or ligaments. These painful areas can move from one area of the body to another, causing the pain to vary from day to day, or they can remain almost constant in certain areas. Because any given area can be closer to nerve endings than another, small swellings can sometimes hurt much more than larger areas of involvement. Pain also varies greatly depending on a person's ability to tolerate it. This seems to be an inherited trait, since we often see patients we can hardly touch, whereas others can be prodded with impunity.

The tender-point concept has always seemed a bit too arbitrary for me. What do we do with someone with all the symptoms of fibromyalgia but who has only nine tender points in the locations we are supposed to check? What if the patient has twenty palpable sore areas in other places, but few among the predetermined sites? Then, as I have just stated, people with high pain thresholds may feel only a little aching, or even no pain at all over the tender-point areas, despite the fact that the doctor can palpate large swollen areas. These patients have all of the fatigue, cognitive, bowel, and urinary tract symptoms of fibromyalgia, but because they do not meet the subjective criteria of pain, they are often diagnosed as having chronic fatigue syndrome.

The concept of tender "points" to me has seemed unduly limiting. My examination finds large and small areas, sometimes entire muscle bundles, that are painful or swollen. For this reason, I prefer to call them the lumps and bumps of fibromyalgia.

❀ WHAT CAUSES FIBROMYALGIA?

The broad spectrum of bodily functions and tissues affected by fibromyalgia make it natural to wonder: What kind of illness could affect so many systems of the body? How can it be so pervasive? Can brittle nails and migraines really be connected? Why can't we find any abnormality on diagnostic tests? These are some of the perplexing issues that physicians and patients alike address and contemplate. Even those of us who have studied fibromyalgia for years do not agree on the answers.

In light of controversies in the medical community about the nature of fibromyalgia, I would like to offer my theory as to what this illness is, and what causes it. Before we delve into its many nuances, please recognize that I am offering this theory based on my personal experience. I have considered and pondered the other proposed theories that attempt to explain the disease. Based on a lifetime of studying the illness and on evidence I have gathered firsthand from more than five thousand fibromyalgia patients, I believe that my theory best explains the problem. It makes the most sense from a physiological and biochemical perspective.

Here I ask the reader to bear in mind that a theory is nothing more than a set of assumptions based on as many facts as can be gathered. When one encounters a theory, he or she should immediately recognize that there are undoubtedly errors and oversights. Ours will surely be improved upon as we learn more about the biochemical mechanisms that I believe are at the root of this illness. So I ask that you please proceed with us patiently. We fully recognize that what follows is *just a theory,* and should be rigorously challenged and tested. We have proven to our satisfaction that fibromyalgia can be treated successfully with our approach. Yet we still aim to find out how and why our medications work—particularly guaifenesin, our most successful treatment to date.

There are those who dispute my assertion that chronic fatigue, chronic candidiasis, vulvar pain, and myofascial pain syndromes, are all names for the same disease. The many symptoms I have described in this chapter are distinctly those of fibromyalgia, but also those of these other diagnoses as well. When physicians extract only certain complaints from patients, the remaining symptoms are ignored. These so-called syndromes come into existence when the elicited complaints are packaged together and labeled.

So above all, I wish we could choose a more descriptive name to fit all the symptoms, which would clarify our treatment approach as well. Fibromyalgia, or pain in muscles and fibers, is clearly inadequate. Chronic fatigue syndrome, the second most commonly used moniker for this illness, focuses mainly on exhaustion. For most patients, both labels apply at various times during their illness. For others, one symptom may always be more prevalent than another. However, when a careful history is taken and a proper examination conducted, it is indisputably clear that both conditions exist simultaneously, although not with the same intensity. This is how we have come to understand that we are dealing with a single condition that presents itself differently, greatly dependent on an individual's pain threshold and on the areas predominantly affected. For this new name, I would use *dysenergism syndrome* (faulty energy) because that ascribes patient fatigue and cellular failure to the same basic metabolic cause. All patients stress that they often cannot muster enough energy to carry out their simple, daily chores. *Anergism* (absence of energy) would effectively describe this lack of vigor in both the struggling patient and the weakened cells. My treatment is designed to restore energy production by releasing the body from a biochemical blockade. When this is accomplished, the symptoms of the illness disappear. Patients who have felt themselves aging rapidly revel in the joy of youthfulness as the good days appear. I can say that in my own case, at seventy I am able to do things I could not do in my thirties.

However much I would love to change the name of our disease, for the purposes of this book we will stick with the name fibromyalgia because it is more practical. We will use it to refer to all the various syndromes and symptoms we have discussed here.

My Theory of the Cause of Fibromyalgia

What is the basic metabolic problem in fibromyalgia that is responsible for all the symptoms we have listed above? Based on the knowledge we have gathered to date, I postulate that fibromyalgia is caused by the retention of a biochemical substance within the cells themselves—a metabolic malfunction that results in an inability to produce energy. This retention begins at birth, and slowly progresses with miniscule accumulations to the point where amounts are sufficient to seriously interfere with normal cellular metabolism. Over time, this accumulation progresses within more and more cells, resulting in an energy deficit, first in certain systems but eventually throughout the body. It is at that point that the disease makes itself known.

Every function of our body needs energy—not only to move, run, exercise, and speak, but also simply to grow hair, breathe, digest our food, fight illness, and especially, to use our brains. Cells utilize a currency of energy, known in biochemical terms as *adenosine triphosphate* (ATP), to perform metabolic chores and the other crucial tasks that are vital to our existence. Energy is very efficiently produced within our cells through extremely complicated biochemical mechanisms. We can identify some of the chemical substances that play integral roles in energy production, one of which would seem likely to be the villain in fibromyalgia. Our observations point to a malfunction caused by an excess of phosphates.

In order to understand how a fibromyalgic's cells malfunction, first let's look at the production of energy in normal individuals. In properly functioning cells, the concentration of phosphate and other substances integral to energy formation is meticulously maintained. Cells use phosphate to produce energy in their power stations, known as the mitochondria. There are mitochondria in all cells of the body, but they are stacked especially high in brain and muscle cells. They are complex little energy factories that convert about eighty percent or more of our foods into the currency of energy, or ATP. (This, you will recall, is adenosine tri*phosphate*—three phosphates hooked on to a single molecule of adenosine.) When a cell must perform a function for the body, it expends one of these high-energy phosphates by tearing it off the adenosine. This action provides almost all of the energy required. Bursts of electrons are released by these and subsequent mechanisms and are almost magically directed to the right place to do the right job at precisely the right time, like plugging in an electric cord. Electrons flow in cells where they run enzymes as electrical current runs appliances. In normal bodies, cells seem to have an almost unlimited supply of ATP. Within thousandths of a second our cells can produce new energy from a reservoir.

So why does an energy deficit occur in a fibromyalgic? We were able to deduce some differences from a study conducted in 1989 that measured ATP levels in fibromyalgics.[8] Two Swedish physicians, Drs. Bengtsson and Henriksson, found a twenty-percent reduction in the level of ATP in muscle biopsies taken from fibromyalgics. They sampled bits of the sore and tender trapezius, a muscle located at the top of the shoulder. In the samples from painful tissue, they found much lower levels of ATP inside cells—and also in their reservoirs, which normally release new phosphates to immediately restore ATP levels as it is used. Normal tissue, which was also biopsied and studied, showed no such ATP deficits. Later, another study found lowered ATP levels in the red blood cells of fibromyalgics. These studies, along with more technical ones (see the

Technical Appendix) support our theory of phosphate retention as the cause of fibromyalgia.

If these studies are valid, as I strongly believe they are, the question immediately arises: What could possibly induce low ATP in cells? Normal ATP levels are essential to all functions of life, and the body is superbly geared to prevent ATP depletion. Obviously, something entering the energy factory is causing a generator malfunction—interfering with the chemical reactions that normally produce ample ATP with ease.

It is well known in physiology and biochemistry that excess phosphate in the inner part of the mitochondria (known as the *matrix*) slows this power station and blocks the formation of ATP because *inorganic* phosphate cannot be converted to a high-energy substance unless it is hooked onto the adenosine molecule. A block in ATP generation means there will not be enough high-energy phosphates available for transport to the cell's action sites. High-activity cells are the first hit and worst affected by this shortage. The more cells are used, the more seriously they are affected. Small wonder that brain and muscles are usually the heaviest hit of all tissues. Cells can function only when their energy is replenished. Is any of this news to a fibromyalgic? This is why I prefer the name dysenergism syndrome to fibromyalgia—because it describes both the obvious fatigue of the patient, and the hidden, biochemical one.

But phosphate is not the only villain. It cannot pile up indiscriminately inside cells without causing permanent damage. Because each phosphate ion carries two negative charges to maintain electrical equilibrium inside the cell, it must be counterbalanced (buffered) by two positive charges. Enter calcium, the main buffer for phosphate. Whenever and wherever excess phosphate builds up in cells, excess calcium does too, and calcium has a very important function inside all cells.

Calcium normally sits quietly inside the cell's storage bin, known as the *endoplasmic reticulum*. When a stimulus arrives, the request for action is signaled to the endoplasmic reticulum, which releases calcium into the main fluid chamber of the cell, the cytosol. The amount released is just enough to perform the desired task, no more and no less. Calcium is the final battery terminal—the ultimate agent that says to a cell: "Do it! Do it!" (See figures 2.1 and 2.2.)

If calcium sparks released from the endoplasmic reticulum goad the cell to action, how does the cell stop its new activity? Calcium does not quit its demands for performance as it sits in the cytosol (known as the *sarcoplasm* in muscles). Whenever calcium is present in the cytosol, the cell is instructed to act and to continue performing until calcium signaling stops. To stop this signal, calcium must be either pumped back into storage within the endoplasmic reticulum, or extruded from the cell. Cells have enzyme pumps that are used just for that purpose. As we already know, any function performed by the body uses ATP as its source of energy, so the enzyme pumps that are used to move calcium out of the fluid chamber also depend on ATP. It has been estimated that forty percent of a cell's energy is expended in moving calcium in and out of storage or out of the cell completely. Since energy needs are poorly met in fibromyalgia because of insufficient ATP, calcium is allowed to sit too long where it is no longer needed. Simply put, there is insufficient energy to fully man the pumps that should bale out the cytosol and dispose of calcium. As a result, tissues affected by the metabolic error that results in fibromyalgia are totally

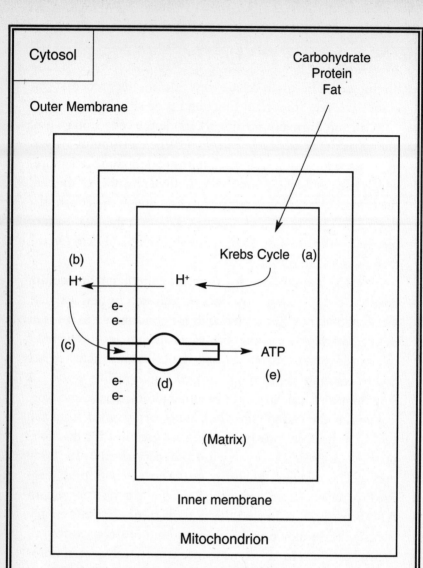

(a) Foods enter Krebs cycle; process releases hyrogen ions (H+).
(b) H+ is driven out to the outer chamber.
(c) H+ enters space within inner wall of mitochondrion and releases electrons (e-).
(d) H+ is driven through proton pump back into the matrix.
(e) Process produces ATP.

Figure 2.1

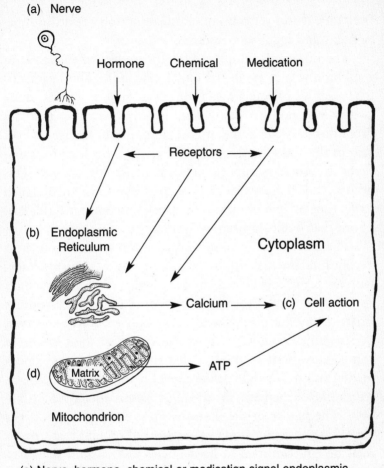

(a) Nerve

Hormone   Chemical   Medication

Receptors

(b) Endoplasmic
    Reticulum   Cytoplasm

                  Calcium ——→ (c) Cell action

(d) Matrix   ATP

Mitochondrion

(a) Nerve, hormone, chemical or medication signal endoplasmic
    reticulum (ER).
(b) ER releases calcium into cytosol.
(c) Calcium initiates cell action.
(d) Mitochondrion produces ATP that provides cell with energy to
    perform whatever it is designed to do.

Figure 2.2

overworked and yet continue in their excessive effort to function day and night to the point of exhaustion.

The numerous lumps and bumps we feel when we examine fibromyalgics are in the muscles, tendons, and ligaments. The areas we palpate are in a contracted state and are working twenty-four hours a day. There is only one thing that can cause this to occur, and that is calcium, out of storage and sitting in the cytosol (sarcoplasm) of a cell. This friend-turned-fiend is providing uncontrolled requests for action. This occurs in all the affected areas of the body. Cells are designed to get time off and proper rest between functions. It is this lack of rest that results in fibromyalgia.

The extent of the fibromyalgic's distress points out how deeply fundamental the basic abnormality is. Patients know without being told that many seemingly unrelated structures are affected. "My whole body is tired; it aches; my bladder is irritated, my gut doesn't work, my brain is addled, and even my fingernails break." I think the extent of these common complaints attests to the fact that the malady is very fundamental and strikes right at the core of living. This widespread, metabolic mayhem can be explained by inadequate ATP function. The nature of the illness is most easily grasped if it is viewed as an accumulation of overworked systems that, true to their design, continue to heed unchecked calcium signals to the point of exhaustion.

We tend to focus on the brain deficits and musculoskeletal pains of fibromyalgia and ignore the very facts confirming that they are victims, just like the rest of the body, of a larger picture. Multiple studies have concluded that there is also a problem within tissues designed for production of molecules, hormones, neurotransmitters, and other chemicals. Most of these are found to be significantly higher or lower, on average, when compared to normal controls. With some variations, researchers have reported low test results for growth hormone; insulin-like growth factor I; serotonin; free ionic calcium; calcitonin; free urinary cortisol; certain amino acids; neuropeptide Y; T cell counts and their faulty activation; and thyroid stimulating hormone response to TRH, which is the normal stimulator.*

On the other hand, higher levels of certain factors are found: prolactin; substance P; angiotensin converting enzyme; and in one study, hyaluronic acid. Skin biopsies have shown disrupted mast cells, which release histamine, among other things (cytokines), under the skin. At these same sites, an excess immunoglobulin G was also found embedded in the deepest skin layers, the dermis. I do not list these scattered and seemingly unrelated findings in order to discuss each abnormality individually or to elaborate on their technical significance. It is simply to illustrate how many different tissues and systems must be affected to alter so many laboratory results. It seems obvious that many new abnormalities will be found in systems already known to be involved. It is also likely that subtler testing will find disorders in tissues we think are unaffected. No matter what is discovered in the future, the lack of ATP would continue to explain the disturbance. If not ATP, I would relish an alternate proposal that could adequately explain the faulty chemistry that I know must exist. Any new theory would need to propose a similar fundamental disturbance serious enough to decimate what was once a smoothly

*These hormones are all defined in the Glossary at the end of this book.

functioning human body. Energy deprivation is certainly at the root of this illness, and only restoration of normal ATP production can reverse this errant metabolism.

Many researchers in the field of fibromyalgia continue to look for a culprit, and another may yet be found. There is certainly more than one gene involved. With women affected far more often than men, the major, defective gene is probably on the X chromosome. We have treated a number of patients under the age of ten, but also many individuals who displayed neither the symptoms nor findings of fibromyalgia until later in life, one at the age of seventy-four. This suggests the presence of one or more less vicious genes. Adding these kinder genes (recessive) to the more harmful (dominant) one permits all types of combinations that would determine how soon in life fibromyalgia is expressed. If both parents have the defect, their children cannot escape it. This would explain the patients we have diagnosed at the age of four, one of whom was already clearly expressing muscle pain by age two.

The human genome will soon be mapped in its entirety, and geneticists will quite likely identify the defective genes in the near future. We strongly suspect that this trait will be coded for a defective enzyme whose job should be to provide perfect phosphate (or other ion) control. This enzyme, or other protein, would normally retain or eliminate phosphate ions with great precision in response to bodily needs. Without it, initially and for a variable number of years, the body is able to tuck away any retained excesses into bones. Though the daily amounts retained are tiny, we believe that eventually this "tuckability" is exceeded, and cellular excessive accumulations begin. For now, however, let's focus on the treatment for reversing fibromyalgia.

Chapter 3

❧

Guaifenesin: How and Why It Works

> I will consider changing my medications, my physical therapies, and even my exercise routine, but I will not consider going without guaifenesin, nor will I take anything that might block its effect. It's too important to my well-being.
> —*Devin Starlanyl, M.D., author of* The Fibromyalgia Advocate

As often happens in medicine, I stumbled upon the treatment for fibromyalgia quite naively, with a patient's chance observation. In 1959, long before fibromyalgia had been defined or given that name, Mr. G suffered from gout and so was taking the only drug available at that time, probenecid (Benemid). He came to my office one day and said, "Hey, Doc, does this medication take tartar off your teeth?" Without much display of social graces, he scraped off bits and pieces of tartar (clinically referred to as dental calculus) and flicked them to my office floor. Though I was not particularly pleased with his uncouth, newly discovered skill, I responded the way a poised physician should. I harrumphed appropriately and said, "I don't think so." Yet my curiosity was piqued, and I began to reflect on this slightly disgusting finding. I awakened during the next two nights asking myself what his flaking prowess might indicate.

Since my knowledge of dentistry was limited, I consulted a dentistry textbook that had a page or two devoted to dental calculus. I found out that tartar contains some trace elements but is made up mainly of calcium phosphate in a chemical structure called "apatite." Tartar develops from saliva, which in turn is derived from the serum of blood. The serum pours out water, all varieties of minerals, proteins, as well as the calcium and phosphate into the salivary glands. The glands manufacture all types of proteins, such as mucus and digestive enzymes, and concentrate the mix to make our saliva. I learned that saliva contains phosphate concentrations four times greater than that of blood. The level of salivary calcium, on the other hand, is about equal to that of blood. Chemically speaking, this is a very unstable solution. Multiplying calcium levels by those of phosphate, a number is derived that we call the solubility constant. When this reaches a certain point, crystals will form and, in the case of tartar, will make deposits on our teeth and under the gum line. Dental calculus can wreak havoc on the gums, teeth, and oral hygiene. That was all the information I could find in that impressive tome. I did know that not everyone's saliva produces dental calculus. Individuals produce tartar at widely varied rates. Some people's teeth are coated with it, while for others it is never a problem. My quest was to learn what was metabolically different about tartar-formers. I began by looking more closely at those with gout, since it was a gout medication that made my tartar-flicking patient such an able performer.

Gout—A metabolic disease unrelated to fibromyalgia. It is diagnosed with a blood test, which will show a high uric acid level. Aspirations of the joint show uric acid crystals. Gout is treated with two types of drugs: uricosuric drugs such as sulfinpyrazone and probenecid, which cause the kidneys to excrete more uric acid, and more commonly now with a drug called allopurinol which inhibits the formation of uric acid. Gout has many symptoms, the most common of which is a red, hot, or swollen joint. It is inherited, and ten times more common in men than in women, where it is usually seen only after menopause.

I had been somewhat fascinated by gout and for a time had suspected that there was more to the illness than merely joint pains and swelling. I reread the original description Thomas Sydenham had written more than three hundred years ago in 1683. He described gout as not only joint pain but also "great mental torpor," "suffusion of the sinuses," generalized flu-like aching and malaise or fatigue, along with many other complaints, all in the dramatic language of his day. In other words, there were systemwide effects which indicated to me that gout was a lot more than just a joint disease.

Uric acid—A waste product from the breakdown of nucleic acids in body cells; also produced in the digestion of some foods. Most uric acid passes by way of the kidneys into the urine and is excreted, although some is passed through the digestive tract. When the kidneys do not excrete uric acid properly, high levels can build up in the blood. This can lead to gout or, to a lesser extent, kidney stones.

Gout is usually inherited, and we know the cause. In susceptible individuals, accumulations of uric acid crystallize and form deposits in the joints. Sydenham's description of systemic symptoms preceding the joint attack made me wonder if there might be a gout syndrome. In this scenario, people would have all of the preliminary symptoms of gout but no joint involvement would follow. Elevated levels of uric acid in the blood would be the cause of this new syndrome. It should also cycle repetitively until, one day, joints would begin to hurt. I thought that perhaps high blood uric acid is able to initiate minideposits in certain tissues such as the brain and the gastrointestinal tract, dust muscles only lightly, and totally avoid the joints until much later in the disease.

I soon found a few patients who had what I thought might be these preliminary gout symptoms: cyclic bouts of fatigue, irritability, nervousness, depression, insomnia, anxieties, loss of memory and concentration. They described generalized, flu-like aching and stiffness mainly in muscles, headaches, dizziness, numbness and tingling of the extremities, and leg cramps as their most prominent complaints. Indigestion with sour stomachs, gas, and flatulence were part of the picture. Our blood tests revealed the anticipated culprit: high blood uric acid (urate). When I treated them with the only antigout medication we had, probenecid, their uric acid levels dropped to normal. I was exhilarated by the fact that their symptoms also disappeared. Oddly enough, although they quickly cleared up, patients relapsed off and on. I noticed, however, that they suffered less intensely and with fewer symptoms during each subsequent attack. We had always known that when we treat gout by lowering the blood uric acid, we precipitated attacks of gouty joints. As uric acid comes out of the joints, it seems to cause the same pains it did going in. My nonarthritic, gouty-syndrome patients also felt all of the same symptoms they had felt before. It was all the same as Sydenham had described except that, I must stress, there was no joint involvement. I realized that those without the joint pains experienced the same thing, a recycling of their symptoms as uric acid was leaving whatever tissues were affected in the first place. This was gout at its best, before there was gout!

Though I was flushed with success, my confidence in my new "gout syndrome without gout" was soon shaken. Here came another group of patients who certainly had all of the symptoms that suggested my new disease. However, they complained of more aches and pains that seemed to come from the entire musculoskeletal system. They had tenderness and swelling in tendons, ligaments, and especially their muscles. Yet no matter how many times I tested their blood, they did not have elevated serum uric acid levels. I decided to put them on gout medication anyhow. They too began recycling the same symptoms as did my elevated uric acid group. Obviously, they were clearing something out of their tissues as well. Gradually, cyclically and progressively, they experienced more good days than bad ones, and ultimately, they went on to complete clearing and remained well as long as they stayed on the Benemid. In short, results were identical in all three groups: those with the classic symptoms of gout, with their red, hot, and swollen joints; those without joint symptoms—the gouty syndrome; and now another condition with no name. One drug was effective against all of these.

This nameless group had many aches and pains, but overwhelming fatigue was just as often their main complaint. I soon realized that women greatly outnumbered the men in this new group. I knew gout was predominantly a male disease and fairly uncommon in women—almost nonexistent in women before menopause. These facts made it ever more likely that there was no connection to gout or the uric acid group except in the similarity of symptoms. My sleeping brain must have been mulling this over since I woke up one night with the thought: "Could there be an entirely new disease that acts like the gouty syndrome and is somehow connected to Mr. G's tartar show? Are there people who retain some other ion (a particle with an electrical charge), other than uric acid, that causes the same bunch of symptoms?"

I found it difficult to stop thinking about this idea, and I began concentrating on patients whose complaints closely mimicked those of the gouty syndrome. Without a named disease (remember, the name "fibromyalgia" has been around only since the 1980s), I had relegated all of these patients, except those with classic gout, to the trash heap of medicine. I would normally have labeled them as my patients with psychiatric problems, my hypochondriacs or my anxiety neurotics. In medicine we had always considered these patients as women who, for whatever reason, suffered from unbalanced hormones, unhappy marriages, empty-nest syndrome, inadequate upbringing, or social maladjustment. When I elicited symptoms somewhat more methodically, I became fascinated by how similar their stories were. If they were suffering from a psychosomatic illness, how could they all invent nearly identical complaints? They didn't know each other; they came from all over the country and from large-scale socioeconomic cross sections of the population. Yet all their symptoms were nearly identical! They cycled with pains, fatigue, and cognitive complaints seemingly without rhyme or reason. In the earlier phases of their disease, they had good and bad days. They were still in the same marriages, had the same children, stress, and fun days, and yet they cycled in and out of their complaints. I knew it was ludicrous to continue in my belief that all of this was due to their nerves, no matter what the books suggested. I knew I might as well accept the fact: there was a real disease, even if it had not been described.

The most common symptoms described by these women were pain, fatigue, emotional and cognitive defects, spastic colon, cramps, numbness and tingling of various parts of the body, and insomnia, which were the same as the gouty syndrome. When I first used the gout medication, probenecid, I met with variable success. The first two patients began the cyclic reversal I had learned to expect in the gouty syndrome. My enthusiasm was soon dashed, however, since I failed with the next three patients. After some initial teeth-gnashing (mine), something told me to try these three failures on a higher dosage. This I did, and the rewards were swift: all three patients began the reverse cycling. It now seemed even more likely that there actually was a tartar syndrome, as I first named it. Equally obvious was the fact that uric acid had no part in the condition, since I could never detect abnormal uric acid levels in these patients. Later I realized that even tartar had no direct relationship to the disease, though it was the change

Mr. G had noticed that first drew my attention. Since tartar was basically composed of calcium and phosphate, one or the other of these seemed a more likely culprit than uric acid.

As I found more and more patients who fitted the mold, I felt certain this was a major illness, far more common than gout, that affected women much more often than it did men. This was a debilitating disease, cyclically but inexorably progressive, and ultimately quite destructive to quality of life. Large numbers of these patients quickly swelled my practice and helped me to expand the parameters of the illness. Soon I realized how often these symptoms seemed to run in families. Older family members related their own horror stories and the litany of their symptoms. The difference was that nearly all of them also had osteoarthritis to contend with as well.

As I worked with these patients, I was touched by their years of suffering, and this further motivated me to refine my treatment. Although the nuances in their stories made each patient a bit different, there was no question that each was ill with the same sickness. One woman spoke of a large area in her back that had been stiff and painful for twenty-four years. Another told me that she hadn't been able to have sex for seven years because of pain and spasm in the vulvar area. Sometimes it seemed I would need a calculator to tabulate the visits to the countless doctors, the tests they had run, and the almost equal number of diagnoses that poured forth. I can repeat a few, but my list is short compared to the real roster. I have heard: "it's a bad menopause," "depression," "inner ear disorder," "defect in your neurotransmitters," "rheumatic arthritis," "migraine syndrome." An army of women were simply told: "It's all in your head; you need a psychiatrist." Some seriously considered suicide, so compromised was the quality of their lives. They were often frustrated and guilt-ridden about not being able to care for their families as they wished. Most of them were acutely aware that they were different from other people without really knowing why. I treated them with probenecid and I achieved significant success in erasing their pain and reversing the general condition.

Some years later, a new uricosuric medication, sulfinpyrazone (Anturane) became available. Later, we found others, such as Flexin and Robinul. All are able to lower uric acid and could work quite well for treating gout. I have used each of them for the gouty syndrome and for our new disease, now known as fibromyalgia. Each of these drugs has only one thing in common: they can each induce uric acid excretion by their action on a certain area of the kidney, the same as does our first drug, probenecid. But remember, fibromyalgia has no connection to uric acid. I feel I must repeat this because of confusion in some circles. It is apparent that since these uricosuric drugs work for fibromyalgia, they must also have another effect on the kidneys. They are obviously clearing something else out in the urine as well.

The metabolic disturbance, then, seemed most likely due to a problem in the handling of either phosphate or calcium. The flaking dental calculus, which some of the women also experienced, provided this clue. I have found that any of the drugs mentioned are capable of slowing or stopping tartar formation, meaning that phosphate or calcium is involved, but it is not a parameter we can monitor because it is so variable. Patients also commonly described chipping and peeling of fingernails in cycles. Nail minerals are predominantly calcium and phosphate just as is tartar. With each attack of what we now call fibromyalgia, new, excessive crystals are laid down at the nail root. As the nails grow out in layers similar to concentric rings of a tree, they chip when the defect reaches the tip. This is why the nails all seem to break at once. Calcium did not seem to be the villain because it actually proved helpful when given with meals as a supplement. We soon found that calcium taken this way permitted us to use somewhat lower dosages of our medications. Calcium binds chemically to phosphate in the intestine, and both are eliminated in the bowel movement. This is good, since less phosphate is presented for absorption and will not flood the system so severely. For these and several other solid chemical reasons, phosphate has remained our main suspect. For further elaboration on these conclusions, please refer to the more technical biochemistry appendix.

Although the drugs we were using to treat fibromyalgia were successful, they did have side effects. Sulfinpyrazone was capable of raising stomach acidity. Probenecid, a sulfa drug, caused allergic reactions in some patients, and Robinul made some patients more tired or slightly spacey. We were always on the lookout for a more effective, easier to tolerate medication. In 1992, more than thirty years after I began my initial research, we got lucky. My nurse's ten-year-old son, Malcolm Potter, had been under treatment for fibromyalgia since the age of seven. As Malcolm grew, we needed larger amounts of his medication, sulfinpyrazone (Anturane), to continue his reversal. As mentioned above, this drug causes hyperacidity and gastric upsets in eight percent of patients. As my young patient grew taller, we were forced to raise his medication to a higher dose, and his stomach started to hurt. We did not wish to try the other medications since they had potential side effects, especially in the amounts he would have required. So we intensified our search for a substitute drug.

We soon found a medication in the *Physicians' Desk Reference* described as capable of minimally lowering uric acid in the bloodstream.[9] It was far too weak to be used in treating gout, but you will recall that any agent capable of lowering such blood levels had proven effective in treating fibromyalgia. We also found a corroborating article in an old copy of the *Journal of Rheumatology*.[10] We stopped his sulfinpyrazone and gave Malcolm guaifenesin. It was an immediate hit, and after knocking Malcolm to the ground with his first reversal cycle, it soon became our star.

Today, guaifenesin is usually an ingredient in cold preparations. But in 1530, in its original form, a tree bark extract called guaiacum, it was in use for rheumatism.[11] It was later also used to treat gout. A paper written in 1928 showed its value for easing growing pains and several other symptoms that now are not difficult to recognize as fibromyalgia. Guaiacum was later purified to guaiacolate, and made its first appearance in cough mixtures about seventy years ago. Over twenty years ago it was synthesized and named guaifenesin, and pressed into tablet form. Its original use, however, is not completely forgotten. In the new *PDR for Herbal Medicines* guaiacum officinale is indicated for rheumatism.[12] The standard dosage for loosening phlegm is two tablets in both the morning and evening (2400 mg per day). In liquid form it is one of the active ingredients in many cough medications, expectorants, and sinus preparations. The drug is no longer under patent and is produced by at least ten different companies, making it widely accessible and affordable. The medication usually comes in a 600 mg tablet and costs about $25 for 100 pills. (Guaifenesin is also available in 300 mg pediatric capsules. These capsules can be swallowed, or opened and the contents sprinkled on food if the child has difficulty swallowing capsules.) Another company is now marketing 1200 mg tablets. Within two hours of ingestion this drug is totally absorbed within the body through the intestinal tract.

Since Malcolm had been off his medicine for some time due to his irritated stomach, we knew we would see something within a few days if guaifenesin were to prove effective. On the second morning after beginning guaifenesin, Malcolm stumbled out of his bedroom exclaiming: "Mom, I can't walk— even the bottoms of my feet hurt!" So pervasive were his

---

Guaifenesin (gwy-FEN-e-sin) is an expectorant that thins mucus and helps to loosen phlegm. Guaifenesin is quickly absorbed from the gastrointestinal tract, and is rapidly metabolized and excreted in the urine. Guaifenesin is also known to lower uric acid levels. No serious side-effects have been reported.[13]

—Physicians' Desk Reference

To read more about guaifenesin, you can ask your pharmacist or doctor for the package insert or consult the *Physicians' Desk Reference* (*PDR*). This is the doctors' guide to medications and has a complete description of guaifenesin. This book can be found in the reference section of libraries, bookstores, or on your pharmacist's and doctor's shelves.

stiffness and aching that we knew we had found a safer and more potent weapon. Since the drug has no meaningful side effects, such an increase in symptoms could only mean we were purging his fibromyalgia. Happily, he was back on the road to recovery.

Why did Malcolm's getting worse signal to us that his FMS was improving? Keep in mind our discussion in Chapter 1 about the lumps and bumps of fibromyalgia. These abnormal lesions we put on a patient's map indicate areas that are tender because they are swollen. Swelling occurs in the tendons and ligaments but mostly in muscles, and these swollen areas press on nerves. Nerves are the only means the body has to transmit messages to the brain. Only the brain can feel pain and then interpret the signals well enough to determine where the problem is located. Ninety to ninety-five percent of the tissue swelling is simply water that has collected under considerable pressure. I suspect the fluid has been lured into cells by the phosphates, calcium, and perhaps other constituents such as sodium. Our bodies send water to these areas in an attempt to dilute the retained ions and to keep them from crystallizing inside the cells. The increased fluid succeeds and keeps the extra accumulations dissolved. This is adequate to permit cell survival, but at the expense of losing some normal cell functions. When each ion has been tucked into the safest storage areas possible, some of the water is allowed to leave and, as the fibromyalgia cycle eases, the bumps seem to get a bit smaller.

When reversal begins, water has to reenter the ailing cells, wherever the purging is to take place. I presume this is necessary to dilute the excess phosphate and calcium concentrations again. The extra fluid, however, again causes swelling and increases pressure, and pain resumes. In other words, the lumps and bumps get bigger at the purging sites. These areas seem under attack all over again. They feel just about the same as they did when fibromyalgia was developing. It feels every bit as bad as it did when deposits were landing in those same tissues before treatment was initiated. It even gets worse than this, since most of the symptoms of the disease resume, not only from the places that are being cleaned out.

When an area is being purged, fluid first accumulates in the cell, as I have stated, but because of the benefits of guaifenesin, it soon reverses its course and withdraws from that same cell. This time, however, it carries out some of the debris, the excess phosphate, calcium, and whatever else that has added to cause the miseries of fibromyalgia. Depending on the amount being pulled from a given site, the bloodstream may suffer varying degrees of flooding by the same debris.

You will recall that I postulate the fibromyalgic kidneys cannot move fast enough when it comes to expelling phosphate. Therefore, the reversal flood is more than they can immediately handle. Since the urine is by far the main route for elimination, the debris pouring out of cells will have to wait its turn to get out of the body. The cell is spring-cleaning and dumps its unwanted phosphate and friends into the bloodstream. This puts an added burden on the blood, which also wants to rid itself of the excess phosphate. It feels for all the world as though the disease were starting all over again, but at its worst level ever, since this purging is moving debris out of cells at least six times faster than the accumulation of the debris. The blood delivers large batches to the kidneys, but those organs cannot process the phosphates instantly. The blood therefore must allow minideposits to occur all over the body, which cause generalized, flu-like aching. The brain scoops up its share, which leads to fatigue, cognitive impairment, irritability, and insomnia. It's déjà vu all over again! The difference this time is that the kidneys are now working in the right direction, thanks to guaifenesin. They are now in overdrive, eliminating the excess phosphate and calcium to the best of their capacity.

The symptoms of fibromyalgia appear to worsen until the kidneys catch up. The main method for eliminating excess phosphates is through the urine. Guaifenesin pulls one batch after another out of the tissues now that the urine is able to eliminate them. These batches obviously contain the disease-causing, accumulated energy blockers. Each cycle ends when that is all that can be done metabolically for the time being. During this leaching out period, patients sometimes notice small amounts of particulate matter in the urine. They also describe unpleasant tastes and odors to their breath, perspiration, and urine. They will notice that their eyes sting and their tears burn.

A rest period then follows, which could last for a few hours, days, or even for weeks if large amounts of the offending substances are being purged. It is likely that the process of reversal is continuing at a subliminal level somewhere even during the better moments. Patients can feel no aching as long as it remains below their particular pain threshold. Suddenly, the crescendo mounts as more cellular debris is stirred up, and the next perceptible attack begins. The patient's individual pain threshold will usually determine the perceived intensity of the reversing attack. Each of these cycles represents a solid step that brings the patient closer to restored health. These reversal symptoms, along with our mapping improvements, have always been our indication that our medications, including guai-fenesin, are highly effective for treating fibromyalgia.

The reversal process can be illustrated with stories told by patients who have been through it.

I have been on guai since mid-October 1998. I took 300 mg twice a day for three months. I felt horrible without letup except for three good days in mid-November. In January, my doctor increased my dosage to 600 mg twice a day. I still felt consistently awful with pain, fatigue, and brain fog until the beginning of the week.

Now I have had a full week of good days. I do admit that when the day is over I am exhausted, but I am sleeping well and am ready to go in the morning. I am glad I did not stop taking the guai because I didn't see results "soon enough." The happiest part for me is that the brain fog has lifted. Now I know that even if I go into flare again, things will get better.

—*Marge W.*

With guaifenesin and our other medications, we have now witnessed benefits from five totally different chemical compounds. Each of these medications has supposedly only one thing in common: the ability to get an area of the kidneys (the proximal tubules) to excrete larger amounts of uric acid. Since uric acid (urate) has no connection with fibromyalgia, we know we are also purging a different biochemical substance. We had measured the urinary output of phosphate, calcium, and urate before and after treatment using probenecid several years previously, and we now retested patients using guaifenesin. We found a sixty-percent increase in phosphate excretion and a lesser one (thirty-percent) in oxalate and calcium with both drugs. But whereas the gout medication significantly increased uric acid excretion, only a minimal increase in urate output occurred with guaifenesin.

The mechanism by which guaifenesin purges the body of phosphate resembles a spigot that drains the kidneys of offending substances. This is analogous to your water system at home. You open the spigot; water flows from your pipes and starts pulling water from the main line. This in turn pulls some water from the entire system, and ultimately the reservoir is lowered by the amount you used in your home, no matter how great the distance between the two locations may be.

Let's now use this analogy to explain my theory—my version—of fibromyalgia. Those of us with one of the defective genes have totally intact kidneys except for one thing. I think there is a defective enzyme that normally would open the spigot wider whenever something accumulates to excess in the bloodstream. I will focus on inorganic phosphate, since that is what I think causes our problem. In chemistry, inorganic phosphate is represented by the symbol, π Pi. Let's use that to simplify my presentation.

The blood brings all sorts of metabolic debris to the kidneys to be filtered into the hollow tubules of the kidneys. This is the beginning of urine. The first flushes have almost identical mineral, chemical, and water concentrations, as the blood does with some notable exceptions. For our purposes, Pi is one of those exceptions. A great deal of this is released all over the body because it is one of the very basic products of energy utilization. Much of it floats downstream. At some point, the cells that line the walls of the tubules in the kidney must make a decision. They respond to the body's needs and either they let all the phosphate go off into the bladder, or if there is the need to retain some, the tubules are capable of reabsorbing the necessary amount of Pi. This system is not quite adequate, however. Fine-tuning is required beyond the capacity of these particular cells at the interface with the new urine. There is such a large amount of phosphate to be excreted that the bottom parts of the cells, away from the hollow tubules, must help.

The bottoms of the cells face capillaries of the bloodstream. Those tiny vessels are able to release more components than the kidney cells can absorb. Pi is one of those substances. The renal cell accepts the substance to internalize it and studies the need to keep it or to reject it by pushing it out of the other side into the urine. These actions are each controlled by different enzymes. I postulate that the reject enzyme is the genetically defective one, but the accept enzyme is another candidate. (We could even speculate that the study enzymes are also defective.) The important conclusion we must come to, to preserve my theory, is that we fibromyalgics cannot pour out enough Pi to keep out of trouble. We cannot open our spigots wide enough to flush all of the accumulating metabolic debris, especially the inorganic phosphate, Pi.

We can set the scene as follows. As cells produce energy, they use a great deal of phosphate. Huge amounts are also needed to control the metabolism of sugar and to build proteins, certain fats, and body structures. The normal wear and tear of cells releases much of this phosphate into the bloodstream, and along with excess coming in from our foods, it is transported to the kidneys. As I have just described, those of us with the faulty spigots cannot quite excrete enough. It is as

Kidney Phosphate Control

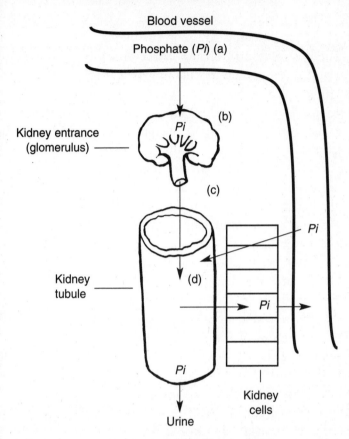

(a) Blood brings inorganic phosphate *Pi* to the kidney.
(b) *Pi* is filtered through the glomerulus and is delivered to the tubule.
(c) *Pi* can also be delivered directly through the blood and through the kidney cells into the tubule.
(d) *Pi* can go two ways from the tubule:
　　　1. Out into the urine.
　　　2. Re-absorbed from the tubule into the kidney cell and back into the bloodstream.
This is how kidney cells "decide" to keep or eliminate phosphates according to what the body needs.

Figure 3.1

though we had a dam downstream and because of this blockage, phosphate attempts to rise in the blood.

The body will not tolerate P*i* accumulation in the blood because it is a *reciprocal* to calcium. This means that if phosphate rises, calcium must drop. The four parathyroid glands in the neck will not permit this. They simply pour out their hormone that serves to maintain calcium levels at all cost. Poor phosphate! It can't escape in the urine and it isn't allowed to hang around in the bloodstream. There is no choice; the tissues must accept some of it back. The bones are the best place for tucking it in, but eventually they can soak up no more. Muscles and sinews must help, and they do. Inorganic phosphate is driven back into cells all over the body. At some point however, this excess slows down the generators, and energy production becomes defective. As we have seen, at this point water enters the cells to dilute the concentration of phosphate and its fellow traveler—calcium—and swelling occurs. The lumps and bumps of fibromyalgia appear, and the whole sequence I have already described is well underway. (See figure 3.2.)

In the first chapter we explained that excess phosphate interrupts normal energy (ATP) production in the cell's mitochondria. If we help our kidneys purge the excess phosphate, our cells will again produce all of the ATP we need. The ATP-controlled pumps will again siphon calcium from where it does not belong and tuck it away neatly into storage. Cells will once again be able to relax, and this rest restores them to the functional, energetic systems they once were. We believe that guaifenesin is the best and safest way to help our enzyme spigots to open wide and let the body get on with its business of metabolism. (See figure 3.3.)

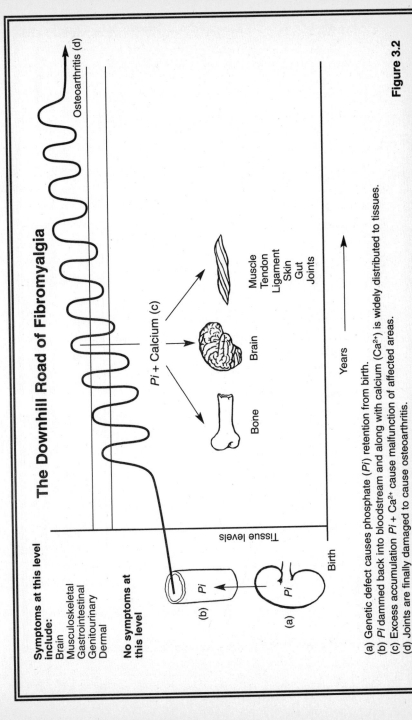

The Downhill Road of Fibromyalgia

Symptoms at this level include:
Brain
Musculoskeletal
Gastrointestinal
Genitourinary
Dermal

No symptoms at this level

Osteoarthritis (d)

Tissue levels

Pi + Calcium (c)

Muscle
Tendon
Ligament
Skin
Gut
Joints

Brain

Bone

Pi (b)

Pi (a)

Birth

Years

(a) Genetic defect causes phosphate (Pi) retention from birth.
(b) Pi dammed back into bloodstream and along with calcium (Ca^{2+}) is widely distributed to tissues.
(c) Excess accumulation Pi + Ca^{2+} cause malfunction of affected areas.
(d) Joints are finally damaged to cause osteoarthritis.

Figure 3.2

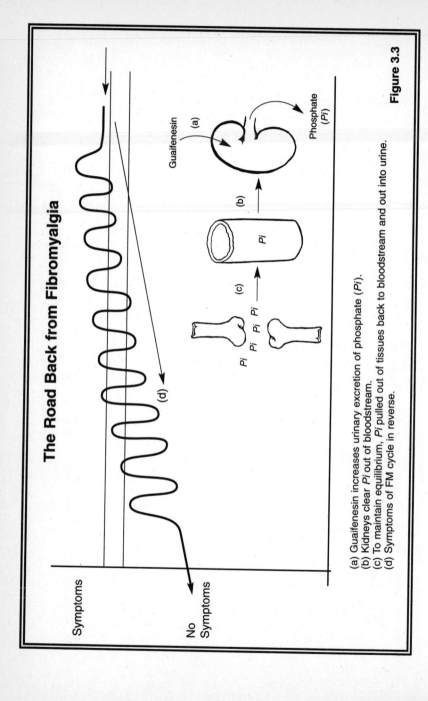

The Road Back from Fibromyalgia

(a) Guaifenesin increases urinary excretion of phosphate (*Pi*).
(b) Kidneys clear *Pi* out of bloodstream.
(c) To maintain equilibrium, *Pi* pulled out of tissues back to bloodstream and out into urine.
(d) Symptoms of FM cycle in reverse.

Figure 3.3

The most difficult aspect of treatment is what patients must go through during reversal. In the early recycling phases, patients are desperate for their bodies to show them even a few good hours. They have been disappointed too many times before by promises of cures that never materialized. We have told them that the first flashes of feeling better will be their assurance of the success to come. If the body is capable of providing them with a few significantly better hours or days, it will be able to do the same on a permanent basis. But until this first glimmer of a healthy future, they can only hope that we have told them the truth and that guaifenesin will work for them as it has for so many others. But the later cycles are hard, too. By then, patients have had a taste of recovery, a series of good days with much less pain and fatigue. So when the next bad cycle starts, they have no idea how long it will last or how bad it will be. At this point, our patients usually express the same concern—they worry that the improved days were only a flash in the pan.

> I started on guai in mid-January 1998. I had experienced FMS symptoms since childhood. I am thirty-four years old and as of January was very ill. I had the gamut of FMS symptoms and was horribly, horribly fatigued and depressed. Now, I am a different woman, only five months later. I am so much better than I have been in years. . . . Fatigue and pain are drastically diminished, and in certain areas I have no pain anymore. Mood has improved. I sleep much better as a rule. My sex life is wonderful. I'm thinking more clearly. Not to say that the road has been easy, no, no, no. Sometimes I couldn't see the light at the end of the tunnel. But

now, it's only five months later and so much is behind me.

—*Julie O., Canada*

Another common reaction is for patients to feel that their body is somehow different from those of all the other fibromyalgics. They have trouble overriding the fear that their case is too far gone ever to get sustained benefits. But as their treatment progresses, their confidence mounts, and relatively soon, patients become old pros at knowing the ins and outs of their disease. They *know* the good days will return in progressively greater numbers. They also learn that attacks will be milder and far more bearable, and fewer and fewer areas will be left to purge. Though the initial reversal cycles might have attacked ten to twenty places at one time, later reversals may work on only one or two sites simultaneously. That alone greatly diminishes the severity of these subsequent attacks. In addition, purging phases get progressively further apart, making these minor setbacks mild by comparison.

Every patient asks: "How long will it take to clear me up?" There is no easy answer. In general, the low-dose person (300 mg twice a day) will go through frequent, almost constant attacks for two or three weeks and suddenly emerge from the other side of the black hole feeling much improved. Dosage is genetically determined, and in a given family, we can fairly well count on the same amount of medication for all its members. The less-responsive patients will need larger dosages and follow a general rule for reversal. We rely on the fact that, in general, for every two months on guaifenesin, we will reverse one year of fibromyalgia. The clock doesn't start ticking however, until we have found the proper dosage, and the patient has totally avoided salicylates. What is most heartening to me is the visible improvement in patients' lives; for some it occurs gradually, as they only slowly overcome their pains, but for others it comes on suddenly—our quick responders.

> I have been on guaifenesin for seven and a half months. I have had painful FMS symptoms since July 1991, following whiplash and a concussion during an auto accident. Since being on guai my quality of life has greatly improved. I have less pain overall, even when cycling. I used to have trouble riding in the car, even for a few miles, because the vibrations felt greatly magnified to me. This has lessened slightly. The severity and frequency of my headaches have diminished significantly. My MPS (Myofascial Pain Syndrome) is gone. I have periods that my skin doesn't hurt when someone touches it lightly, I used to hurt all the time from a soft touch or rub. I am capable of doing much more day-to-day things like loading the dishwasher and watching our children during the day. I need to rest quite a bit less. . . . I have had a full three weeks with virtually no pain. This is the first time in seven years that this has happened. This treatment is our one great hope.
>
> —*J. M., Texas*

Another patient who went through years of hardship with fibromyalgia, and had difficult cycling during treatment, recounts her experience:

I want to brag about my second thirty-mile bike ride. I am very proud of myself. I want you to know how far I've come. I am forty-eight years old and suffered all my life with progressively more and more pain and depression. I have been on most of the powerful painkillers and antidepressants over the years. I closed my business and quit working in 1994. My mind was worthless, the fatigue and pain made getting out of bed impossible on most days, and I had horrid insomnia for years. The symptoms would come and go, and most of the time I "looked normal," although I put on a lot of weight. Life has always been a fight against body and mind pain. In February of 1997 I was hit hard. My entire body swelled, my skin burned all over, my mouth burned badly and I salivated constantly. My stomach contorted. My mind went crazy. Most of my muscles were in spasm. I couldn't move without sweating profusely.

—*G. W., Los Angeles*

Before we end this chapter and leave the subject of guaifenesin, I'll take a moment to answer the most commonly asked questions about guaifenesin:

Does guaifenesin have side effects?

Other than rare nausea (usually transient), guaifenesin has no known side effects. If you are one of the rare individuals who gets an upset stomach on the medication, simply break the tablet in half and put it into a gelatin capsule (purchase at a pharmacy or health food store). The stomach cannot digest gelatin. This allows the capsule to slip into the small intestine before it is broken down. The commercial guaifenesin capsules contain only 300 mg and are far more expensive than the tablets. Very rarely, patients have an allergy to one of the fillers or dyes in the tablets and, in very rare instances, to the guaifenesin itself. For patients sensitive to the dyes, or chemically sensitive patients, a white (dye-free) guaifenesin tablet is on the market. Even occasional hives or other rashes seem to be mostly due to purging the fibromyalgia from the skin. The pain, numbness, and the host of other symptoms you feel while taking guaifenesin are due to the reversal process itself. They are your best clues that the guai is working. Thus feeling worse means you're getting better.

Which guaifenesin should I use?

Guaifenesin is an ingredient in many cough mixtures and decongestants, but these are not good sources of the medication and should not be used to treat fibromyalgia. Any pure guaifenesin that has no added pseudoephedrine, dextromethorphan, or any of the other compounds that may cause side effects is recommended. Liquid guaifenesin preparations are inappropriate because of the low dosage and the sugar, sorbitol, alcohol, or dye contents.

Can I get guaifenesin over the counter?

Guaifenesin is available in 200 mg tablets over the counter, but I do not recommend self-treatment. Fibromyalgia is best diagnosed and treated by a medical doctor. It is sometimes difficult to find the correct dosage, especially in the early stages when symptoms get worse. That is very trying for patients, a time when they will need medical assurance. The many symptoms of fibromyalgia could easily mask some other condition and may therefore require the input of a physician before and during initial treatment. It could be dangerous to assume all symptoms are due to FMS. It will also be important as treatment progresses to have a doctor who is knowledgeable about FMS and its reversal. It may take a professional to discover that some salicylate is blocking guaifenesin. There are times when a patient may need to be reevaluated, since another illness could creep in.

Are there any special instructions for storing guaifenesin?

The medication should be stored in an area that has a temperature between 59 and 86 degrees Fahrenheit, not in the refrigerator or in a very warm room.

My prescription says I need to drink lots of water with my guaifenesin. Is this true?

Many prescriptions for guaifenesin will come with this instruction on the label. This suggestion is placed there for patients who are taking guaifenesin for lung or sinus problems. The extra fluid intake further helps to loosen mucus. It is not necessary for fibromyalgics to increase their intake of water while on guaifenesin.

Who profits from the sale of guaifenesin?

The companies that manufacture it, which are, by and large, generic houses. It is no longer under patent, and over ten companies make it. This is why it is inexpensive. Pharmacies add to their profit as well.

Should I continue my other medications when I start guaifenesin?

Typically, your doctor will allow you to continue all other medications except those that contain aspirin, which will block guaifenesin at the kidney level, rendering it useless for fibromyalgia. (It will still liquefy your mucus.) For example, you must avoid Soma Compound (replace with plain Soma), Darvon Compound (replace with Darvocet-N), Fiorinal, Percodan, and Empirin. Some of these preparations are made with Tylenol instead of aspirin and each exists as a cheaper, generic product. You will also have to discontinue some over-the-counter medications such as Pepto-Bismol, which contains salicylic acid (see Chapter 4).

Some people refer to the guaifenesin protocol as detoxification. Is that correct?

There are no toxins in fibromyalgia. In all the extensive testing done on fibromyalgics, no toxins have been found. Whatever is causing FMS, it is a normal body constituent that the body does not regard as an enemy. There is no inflammatory response, and there are no antibodies to whatever it is. Since there are no toxins, guaifenesin does not "detox."

Is it beneficial to cleanse the body of yeast and/or parasites before starting guaifenesin treatment?

We normally do not see FMS patients with these conditions and thus put our patients on guaifenesin without the hugely expensive tests necessary to detect these problems. Also, the diagnoses of systemic yeast overgrowth or parasites are not always reliable. Remember that in fibromyalgics the immune system is depressed, which can quite often result in recurrent yeast infections in women. You will note that the candida, or yeast, diet is quite similar to the one we use for hypoglycemia.

Is guaifenesin safe to take if I get pregnant?

Guaifenesin is actually used to help women get pregnant—it liquefies the mucus plug that normally sits at the opening of the uterus. We suggest each woman discuss this issue with her own doctor. We advise our pregnant women to stop and, with the permission of their obstetrician, resume treatment after the six month of pregnancy. The baby is fully formed by that time. This way the woman avoids the sudden burst of symptoms that quickly follow delivery.

Am I at greater risk of osteoporosis when taking guaifenesin?

The calcium excreted by guaifenesin is limited to the inappropriate calcium surplus in your cells. So you don't have to worry about the calcium excretion causing osteoporosis.

Can guaifenesin cause kidney stones?

No, there is no connection between kidney stones and guaifenesin. Most stones are calcium oxalate, some are sodium urate, and a smaller number are calcium phosphate. Guaifenesin has been in use for many years and has never been linked to kidney stones. There is also no connection between kidney stones and fibromyalgia.

Is it O.K. to drink colas while taking guaifenesin?

We have not had to restrict colas when we treat fibromyalgia. They do contain phosphoric acid, and phosphate is the ion we are trying to purge from the body, but the amount of phosphate in soda is minute. Guaifenesin appears to overcome that small, added load rather easily as it also overcomes the tiny amounts that are contained in nearly all of our foods.

If I have asthma, can I take guaifenesin?

Actually, guaifenesin is frequently used in asthmatics. It's on the market as a "mucolytic" agent, something that liquifies mucus. It therefore helps to loosen mucus and make it easier to raise. So it may end up helping your asthma. But if you have any medical conditions such as asthma, you should always consult with your own doctor. This book is designed to help you and your doctor understand and successfully use the guaifenesin protocol. It is not meant to take the place of your own doctor.

And now, let's move forward and learn more about the protocol. The next few chapters will tell you more of the things you will need to know about guaifenesin and fibromyalgia.

After the initial onslaught of the illness, there was disbelief. I sat in my chair for hours not believing I could possibly be living in such a broken body. The pain came in waves, rendering life an unpredictable nightmare of perceived uselessness and anger. I gave up my role as a wife, a mother, a daughter and a therapist. I had loved each of those roles. [The depression began] so long ago I don't even remember. I prayed to God. Then I quit praying. No strength for it. I gave in and gave up and spent most of the time doing nothing. It is so easy to get stuck right there doing nothing, not caring, not wanting to live, hoping not to die. It is hard work to be sick. It's harder work to get well . . . but getting well is the best thing there is, and guaifenesin is the way to do it.

—*Gretchen, South Carolina*

Chapter 4

❦

Know Thine Enemy: Salicylates

❦ MEET THE ENEMY: ASPIRIN AND OTHER
SALICYLATES, NATURAL AND OTHERWISE

A Brief History of Salicylates

Guaifenesin, our star drug for treating fibromyalgia, has one
and only one enemy that completely blocks its effectiveness. Its
foe is a chemical compound known as salicylate.[14] All plants
produce it as a protective agent against soil bacteria. Without
salicylates, plants would never get out of the ground alive.
Today, salicylates are easily made synthetically in laboratories,
so salicylates exist both as natural and synthetic compounds.
The best-known and most commonly used salicylate is good
old aspirin, acetyl*salicylic* acid, which is synthetic.

Salicylates have been used medicinally for at least 2000
years. In the fifth century B.C., Hippocrates, the father of medicine, used a juice extracted from the bark of willow trees to

treat aches and pains. Other cultures, such as the American Indians, used meadow grass and tree barks for the same purposes, from which they prepared topical preparations and medicines that were taken internally. During the late Middle Ages, the willow-bark concoction was so popular in Europe that it had to be outlawed. So many people were stripping the bark and killing the trees that the wicker industry—which needed the same trees to make furniture—was nearly destroyed. In 1806 the law was repealed in desperation because Napoleon's blockade of the continent had halted the importation of Peruvian quinine, the only alternative drug. This greatly renewed interest in willow bark inspired chemists to successfully isolate salicin, the active ingredient for pain relief.

Scientists from Italy, Germany, and France competed to make a stable synthetic compound they could market. This was finally accomplished in 1893 by an industrial chemist named Felix Hoffman whose father had severe arthritis and could not tolerate natural medicines. This man-made salicin was called acetylsalicylic acid (ASA) and was given the trade name Aspirin, which we still use today. It was introduced to doctors in 1899 as a commercial prescription drug. In 1915 it became available to the public as an over-the-counter medication. By the 1920s and thirties, aspirin had come into widespread use for fever, rheumatism, lumbago, and neuralgia.

Aspirin has extensive effects on the body. We all know it as an effective pain-reliever, especially for arthritis, backache, and headache. Aspirin works by reducing the body's ability to form prostaglandins, compounds that induce inflammation. Aspirin also reduces the risk of heart attacks and strokes by lessening the chances of blood clots. It accomplishes this by making the platelets, the elements of the blood that initiate clots, less likely

to stick together. It is often used following heart attacks to reduce damage. Aspirin may help prevent certain types of cata-
racts as well as affording some protection against colon and
rectal cancers. In its concentrated form, salicylic acid is used to
remove warts and corns. The acid is also commonly used for
treating acne and dandruff. Many skin products contain this
acid as well, listed as betahydroxy acid (BHA). Women often
unknowingly use the agent as an ingredient in their facial
cleansing creams, where it provides an exfoliating action and
removes dead skin.

The word "natural" on product labels has become the
major sales gimmick of the nineties. Suddenly and increasingly, the value of a product today seems for many people to
lie in how natural it is. Because of this, natural salicylates in the
form of plant parts are commonplace ingredients in many of
the products we use every day. These include shampoos, conditioners, cosmetics, topical creams, herbal remedies, muscle
balms, toothpastes, deodorants, cough drops, suppositories,
and many more products sold under countless trade names.

The ingestion of salicylates by Americans has increased
dramatically in the past decade. They are sometimes used as
food preservatives and are often found in artificial colors and
flavorings. Salicylates are fairly praised for their usefulness and
therapeutic benefits. For fibromyalgics being treated with guaifenesin, they are not only a detriment but are also our arch-
enemies! There are other people who must avoid salicylates as
well—they are a common allergen and have been presumed to
be a cause of Attention Deficit Disorder (ADD) and other
problems in sensitive children. There is a nationwide organization known as the Feingold Association, named for the doctor who postulated the connection, which is a valuable

resource for children and their families who must avoid all salicylates for the above reasons.

Why Salicylates Block Guaifenesin

How can salicylates have such a deleterious effect on guaifenesin treatment? The answer is not very complicated. There is a
particular area in the kidneys where guaifenesin, as well as our
previously successful medications, must be allowed to work
unimpeded. Unfortunately, it is precisely the same location
where salicylates also attach. All biological cells have surface
areas that house thousands of receptors. Think of each receptor as a little garage. Each garage will allow parking for only the
best chemical fits. Each receptor is precision-made to accommodate only specific hormones or chemicals. For any medication to work, it must find and fit into a garage, even though
the space was intended for a natural molecule. This is what the
science of pharmacology is all about. Drugs are manufactured
to occupy natural receptors that will either trigger an action or
have a blocking effect. Once medications are correctly parked,
cells under their influence will perform or not perform specific
actions. The proximal renal tubule is where the receptors are
located that permit access to guaifenesin. Unfortunately,
salicylates are elite competitors for these same receptors and fit
better in those spaces than guaifenesin or any of our other
medications. It takes very little salicylate to occupy the few
available sites, and this will leave no room for guaifenesin.
None of the drugs we have used, regardless of the quantity, can
overcome this discriminatory behavior by the receptors in the
kidneys. In the presence of even small amounts of salicylates,

the parking lot is closed to guaifenesin. The drug will still liquefy mucus, but its benefits for fibromyalgia will be zero.

We have labored with this problem of blockage for many years now. We knew to avoid aspirin from the very beginning because it is well known to stop the action of all uricosuric drugs at the kidney level. As we went along, we were crushed when we began to learn the many hidden sources of salicylates and how easily they are absorbed through the skin. Their pervasive presence is so overwhelming that, at times, I feel paranoid about what seems like a personal assault on our patients by the herbal medication and cosmetic industries.

A number of studies have demonstrated how effectively salicylates are absorbed through the skin and then widely distributed by the bloodstream throughout the body. In one such study, doctors rubbed a pain-relieving cream into the trapezius, a muscle at the top of the shoulder area. One and a half hours later, biopsies were taken from that muscle and from the one on the opposite shoulder.[15] Salicylate levels were nearly identical in both, even though the cream was rubbed into the skin on only one shoulder. (Please refer to the Technical Appendix for a more detailed discussion of the blocking action of salicylates.)

> I have suffered with FMS symptoms since 1991. I began on guaifenesin just a short time ago. Since Dr. St. Amand has taught me about salicylates, I have discovered that not only do they block guaifenesin, they have had a harmful effect on me throughout my life. I was always into natural products. I owned a natural food store and used herbal products inside and out for years. I

could never understand why so many others were so healthy and I (the owner) was constantly sick with one thing after another. Having always been quite level-headed and easygoing, I found myself turning into a raving lunatic as time went on, and finally sold my business, racking it all up to stress.

After about a year of getting away from these products, I started to settle down and didn't have as many physical ills. So I started working again as a florist and garden landscaper. Sure enough, I became very ill again both emotionally and physically. I never put two and two together, I just thought I was allergic to working. Looking back over the last two years, I noticed that every time I worked outside in the dirt and plants, I got very ill with all the same symptoms and ended up in bed for two to three weeks.

After reading the information Dr. St. Amand provided, I finally found out what had been happening to me. I immediately weeded out all salicylate products and started using gloves if I was outside touching anything around the dirt and plants. I believe with all my heart that Dr. St. Amand has truly found the key to all our pain and suffering.

—*Jayne W., FL*

Some physicians scoff at my insistence that topical salicylates can readily block guaifenesin. To this I say: Nonsense! I am the only one with the experience and documentation to confirm what I say. I have made hundreds of maps that illustrate all too well the complete reversal of previous improvement in patients when salicylates were introduced in any form.

Ignore any and all voices to the contrary. Salicylates block with devastating efficiency. Sensitivity to blockade is genetically determined and, since none of us knows our personal susceptibility, each should meticulously abide by the protocol. There is no need to belabor this point. To our fibromyalgic readers I plead—do your job and give guaifenesin a fair chance. Do not improvise on your own by altering our warnings. A little dab of something can totally block your chances of recovery, and you will think we failed you!

Avoiding Salicylates

Since my first day in medical school, I have had a love affair with medicine. Our relationship had never been close to shattering. That is, not until it was severely strained by my almost-daily torment of trying to guess the new, hidden source of salicylates blocking a particular patient. I spend much time cautioning patients on how to avoid various sources beyond simply not taking aspirin and Pepto-Bismol. Even our best efforts have not prevented errors too frequently committed by intelligent and diligent people. The inability to use a beloved product from the beauty shelf seems heart-wrenching for some people, and the most difficult part of their treatment. Others, however, will give up anything without a second thought for a chance to get well.

My first visit with a new patient usually proceeds well when I take a history, complete my examination, and produce my map of the patient's lesions. Then I make a sketch as I tell the patient a story—our version of fibromyalgia. I run through the details of how we began, thanks to the observant man with flaking tartar. We flit superficially through the metabolism of calcium and phosphate as I believe it relates to fibromyalgia. We dwell a bit longer on the cyclic but progressive nature of the illness and on its genetics. I spend considerable time explaining the role of guaifenesin in reversing our warped chemistry and the starring role of the kidneys in the disease. Patients grimace a bit when I describe the ritual dance of the reversal process. I tell them it is natural to expect great swings in symptoms, which cycle rapidly from worse-than-ever to better-than-in-a-long-time hours and then days. The dance is fascinating for all but those who must participate. Patients handle this information quite well—so far so good.

It is almost certain that I will get the worst verbal or facially expressed protests when I come to the matter of herbal preparations. Since eighty-five percent of our fibromyalgics are women, to ban the use of their favorite beauty products is like asking them to commit cosmetologic suicide! We have actually had a few patients dump guaifenesin and me rather than give up cherished items. Believe it or not, we have actually heard: "I'd rather have fibromyalgia than give up my lipstick!" It is sometimes equally difficult to convince patients to part with their all-natural herbal megavitamins and echinacea or ginkgo-biloba. At that point I gracefully suggest that had these herbal supplements reversed their fibromyalgia, they would not be sitting in my examination room listening to me.

Why will herbal medicines block guaifenesin while cooking herbs will not?

Herbal medicines are made from plants. The chaff is removed, leaving the choice parts that contain the most salicylate and are often made even stronger by distillation. Food plants, because they are not concentrated, contain only small amounts of salicylate that when eaten are first directed to the liver. The liver adds either glycine or glucoronide to the salicylate, which renders the compound even less potent. Larger salicylate bursts, as caused by herbal medications, overwhelm the liver and deliver the naked compound directly to the kidneys. The same principle holds true for herbal teas. Commercial herbal teas that are used for hot beverages will not block guaifenesin. Medicinal teas from health food stores are concentrated for medicinal purposes and are therefore too high in salicylates for guaifenesin users.

It is easy to avoid acetylsalicylic acid, aspirin. Pain medications of many types contain this drug, which becomes salicylate when it enters the body. It is slightly more difficult, however, to avoid salicylate when it is blended into a chemical marriage such as octylsalicylate, found in many sunscreens; bismuth subsalicylate (Pepto-Bismol) or methyl salicylate in Listerine and Bengay. Recovery demands that patients learn to read labels and grasp the nature of each ingredient in a product.

Cosmetics, lotions, vitamins, and supplements sold in the United States must, by law, list all of their ingredients, at least on some part of their packaging. Sometimes the individually wrapped products such as lipsticks or eye pencils you find in stores will not list the ingredients because they were listed on the larger container in which they were packaged. For these you will need to find the original packaging the store received, or contact the manufacturer directly. In products such as lip balms, it is common to see a listing for "active ingredients."

The inactive ingredients are not listed, and these are the ones that pose a problem for us. When aloe or an herb is added to these compounds, they are usually considered to be inactive ingredients. Again, the manufacturer or retailer will have to help supply the missing information. Guaifenesin users get the splendid opportunity to become salicylate sleuths and amateur botanists. They must remain vigilant, because manufacturers change ingredients without warning, almost daring you to find the hidden blocker. (Is my paranoia showing?)

> **How do I know if a product contains herbs or salicylates?**
> You must read the labels of everything you use on your skin, even lipsticks and razors. The complete list of ingredients is sometimes found only on the original package. You may have thrown it away when you bought the product. If it came packaged in bulk, the store may have thrown the larger box away. If the label is vague or incomplete, with such statements as "active ingredients" or "other ingredients," you will need to look farther. You may be able to get complete information only by calling the manufacturer, but when in doubt, *do not use the product.*

When those on guaifenesin buy a replacement product, it is necessary to recheck the label, each and every time. This game must be replayed regardless of the number of times you have purchased the identical merchandise or how long you may have used it. It is not uncommon to find two bottles of the same product sitting next to each other on the grocery store shelf, one containing aloe, and the other containing none. Sometimes manufacturers are helpful and add a little banner reading, "Now with ALOE and GINSENG," but you cannot trust them to do this routinely.

Sources of Salicylates

NATURAL SALICYLATES

I am deliberately repetitious but, when taking guaifenesin for fibromyalgia, it is imperative to avoid *all* sources of salicylates. It will not suffice to avoid just *some,* regardless of whether or not they are natural or synthetic. Natural salicylates are becoming more and more common in the form of herbal medications. Many of these have now made the popularity charts and best-seller lists and are commonly believed to perform all sorts of miracles. When properly prepared, these bits and pieces of plants do some of the things they are advertised to do, but their salicylate content is sufficiently potent to totally block guaifenesin—which is what we're concerned with here.

In addition, it seems appropriate to question the wisdom of ingesting over one hundred thousand compounds simply to get to a couple of effective ones. It also bears mentioning that dietary supplements, cosmetics, and herbal concoctions are not required to meet the standards of the Food and Drug Administration (FDA). The quality of supplements is up to the manufacturer, and not all of them are honorable or even careful. Batches of herbs are often imported from Third World countries where they may have been grown and harvested in questionable surroundings and treated with unknown chemicals. Scientific studies done on these herbal supplements have shown a wide variability in the potency and content from manufacturer to manufacturer and from batch to batch. Therefore, claims made on cosmetic packaging and medicinal herbs are merely advertising slogans, and should be viewed as such.

While taking guaifenesin, it is not necessary to avoid the salicylates contained in our foods. Even those with greater salicylate content, such as berries, fruits, vegetables, cooking herbs, and spices, do not block guaifenesin. The ingested compounds are partially destroyed by digestive processes and further altered by the liver. Salicylate levels can be measured in the blood and in the urine and the average daily intake from foods are in the range of 10 to 20 mg. It was once speculated that increased ingestion of salicylates from foods might explain the lower incidence of heart attacks witnessed in recent years. This has been refuted. A recently reported study tested urinary salicylate levels resulting from various diets. It proved previous conventional wisdom correct: foods add insignificant amounts of salicylate to the urine and, presumably, to the bloodstream. We have seen no guaifenesin blockage from any foodstuffs and we impose no dietary restrictions on patients who have only fibromyalgia. However, if you are a fibromyalgic and your symptoms fit those discussed in the chapter on hypoglycemia and fibroglycemia, you are in a situation where a diet is all-important for improvement.[16]

The salicylate content of many foodstuffs has been tested for research on food allergies, and researchers have found that not all parts of all plants contain salicylates. Oatmeal is one such plant part, which is why persons taking guaifenesin may use some of the oatmeal-based Aveeno products, for example. However, it is much better to err on the side of caution when in doubt. Although the kernels of grains (wheat, oats, barley, and rye) contain no salicylate, this is not the case for the rest of the plant on which they grow. Thus wheat kernels are free of salicylates, but wheatgrass and other parts of the wheat plant do contain them. Articles showing the salicylate content of various foods can be found on the Internet or in medical journals. Patients should bear in mind that since salicylate content varies from plant to plant, the numbers in these studies should not be considered one-hundred-percent accurate.[17]

Single chemicals extracted from plants, other than salicylate itself, are acceptable and will not block guaifenesin. For example, alpha-hydroxy, or fruit acid, does not contain whole plant parts, and will not block guaifenesin. Other ingredients in this category are: cetyl alcohol, stearic acid, stearyl alcohol, acetic acid, sodium cocyl isethionate, oleoresin, cocamidopropyl, caprylic triglycerides and glycerides, capric acid, beta-carotene, shea butter, cocoa butter, coconut fatty acids, starch, and hydrogenated soy glyceride. In the same way, bromelain, an enzyme isolated from papaya and used to aid digestion, will not block guaifenesin. If it sounds more like a chemical than a plant, or is a single enzyme or chemical isolated from a plant source, it is acceptable for use with guaifenesin.

Plant ingredients in most products are not difficult to identify. Rose hips, lavender, rosemary, ginseng, chamomile, and aloe vera are some of the well-known ones. Less commonly known names such as arnica, jojoba, and yucca can be identified with the use of a regular dictionary.

Which dishwashing liquids are salicylate free?
Dish soaps are usually fine except for some found at health food stores. Those may contain herbs or seed oils.

There is, unfortunately, another group of plant names that are impossible to find in any standard reference books. Since the basic ingredients in all cosmetics are similar, manufacturers search for unique sounding additives that will set their product apart on labels and in advertisements. Rainforests and tropical islands are being raided for cajeput, quillaja, bibia, padauk, and other native plants. These exotic but obscure substances can sometimes be identified only by searching in a dictionary of cosmetic contents, such as Ruth Winter's *A Concise Dictionary of Cosmetic Ingredients*. However, even this excellent reference work cannot keep up with the cosmetic companies' rainforest scavengers, who are eager to find something that is reasonably safe and will make their product stand out from their competitors. You must call the manufacturer and, with a bit of luck, you can learn if the funny name on the product label is actually a plant. You should also be aware that there are occasional ingredients that are almost mystical since no one seems to know what they are or is unwilling to tell. Sea silt is one of those. It should mean dirt if it is silt, but what else crept into it? Does it come from the ocean bottom or simply from some beach, and does it, then, contain plant parts, too? There is no way for us to have any idea of the salicylate content of something like that. Such products should be avoided in order to give the guaifenesin and especially you, the patient, a fair shake.

Ingredient dictionaries are important for all patients who switch products and use a variety of substances on their skin or hair. Only with such a dictionary is one able to know, for example, that vanilla is a plant and vanillan is artificial, and that anise is a plant and anisole is synthetic.

Attesting to the skin's ability to absorb chemicals, every few years another prescription medication is approved by the FDA for transdermal use. These medications are usually put in a patch that is applied to the skin. From there they are absorbed directly into the bloodstream. A current list would include hormones, analgesics, and narcotics, as well as chemicals such as nicotine. The benefit of delivering these and other substances directly into the bloodstream is that it permits the use of smaller dosages because the medication does not have to pass through the digestive system. Some side effects such as stomach upset can be avoided as well. This fact alone should alert patients to the fact that the skin surely provides a receptive surface for the absorption of many compounds. I think this should frighten us all, more than just a bit. We so happily inflict upon ourselves tubes and jars full of substances in our zeal for youthful skin and dazzling beauty. Yet what else does the skin absorb from the botanical garden enclosed in these bottles, along with the preservatives needed to keep them from spoiling?

Lipsticks, lip balms, mouthwashes, deodorants, muscle balms, suppositories, chewing gums, over-the-counter medications, nasal sprays, breath mints, toothpastes, razors, and shaving creams have the potential to block guaifenesin. Some of these products contain camphor or castor oils; others add natural flavors such as mint, spearmint, peppermint, or wintergreen oils that, in susceptible individuals, will provide enough salicylate to block guaifenesin. Manufacturers have added a strip of aloe behind the cutting edge of most women's disposable razors. This aloe, which spreads onto the myriad of tiny cuts made by shaving the legs and under arms can easily block guaifenesin. Some hair sprays are proud to list aloe or a variety of herbs to spritz onto your hair, but they also land on your scalp and forehead. At first glance it may seem we are

being picky, and that the amount of salicylate in these substances is very small. These items are on our list because each
has blocked several of our patients who had made an early
improvement but suddenly regressed. I wish we could send
each of them a letter of deep appreciation for their teaching
skills.

> *I'm a gardener. Is there anything I should be careful about?*
> You should be very careful doing certain gardening
> chores. Plant saps are readily absorbed through the skin.
> You should wear gloves if a particular job will expose you
> to plant juices. The thin latex variety of gloves worn by sur-
> geons are ideal for delicate tasks, while thicker, leather-
> palmed gloves should be worn when doing heavy work.
> Plants such as mint, marigold, geranium, and rosemary
> have higher salicylate contents than others. However, it is
> best to assume that all plants can block guaifenesin.

We are also concerned about the amount of salicylate that
is inhaled into the bronchial tree by smokers, including marijuana users. We do not know the full impact of this as yet. We
do know from experiments with tobacco plants that tobacco
leaves make methyl salicylate. They are treated, hanged, and
dried, but that alone would not destroy our offender. The possibility exists that smoking could make guaifenesin partially or
totally ineffective. It might merely depend on the crop's potency, but we ask patients to become as pure as possible and to
avoid any substance they cannot *totally* validate. *Any product is
suspect until one can obtain proof that no botanicals or salicylates
have been added.*

Despite protests, it is critical that guaifenesin users fully comply. Without any doubt, our greatest cause of treatment failure is patient noncompliance or ignorance (our own included) in identifying such blockers.

Common Medications Containing Natural Salicylates
(The offending substances are listed in parentheses)

Aloe Vera

Celestial Seasonings Throat
  Drops (chicory root and
  anise)

Dhea Plus (gingko-biloba)

Dong Kwai

Ephedra

Feverfew

Gas-X (mint oil)

Gingko-Biloba

Naxixx (Chinese herbs)

Pau D'Arco

Preparation H Ointment
  (thyme oil)

Purge (castor oil)

St. John's Wort

Saw Palmetto

Valerian

Vicks Cough Drops
  (eucalyptus oil)

Common Topical Preparations Containing Natural Salicylates
(The offending substances are listed in parentheses)

Absorbine Jr. (calendula,
  echinacea, wormwood)

Aloe Vera Gel

Arthricare

Cortaid Maximum Strength
  Cream (aloe vera gel)

Dolorac Cream (capsicum)

Gum and Toothache
  Medications (clove oil)

Hemorid (aloe barbadensis
  extract)

Milk of Magnesia (cascara)

Vaseline Intensive Care Sunless
  Tanning Lotion (aloe)

Vicks Vaporub Cream
  (eucalyptus oil)

Zostix Cream (capsicum)

SYNTHETIC SALICYLATES

The synthetic offenders are easier to avoid than are the natural ones because the word salicylate, salicylic acid, or the syllable "sals" will be in the ingredient list on the label. There are many medications used for pain relief or to reduce inflammation, such as salsalate. Other compounds include sodium salicylate, choline salicylate, and magnesium salicylate. Aspirin may be listed on labels as ASA (a common designation for acetylsalicylic acid), although this is more common in Canada than in the U.S. You may also see choline magnesium trisalicylate, or salicylsalicylic acid. A glance at this list of names will quickly show the syllable "sal" in each compound. Overzealous patients have often confused this syllable with "silica," a mineral often found in cosmetics that will not block guaifenesin.

Synthetic salicylates are also present in mouthwashes, where they are listed as salicylic acid or methyl salicylate. It has recently come to our attention that most toothpastes contain salicylates, either as unlisted salicylic acid or as methyl salicylate, identified on the label only by the word *flavor.* For this reason patients must use a nonmint toothpaste. Tom's of Maine makes two children's toothpastes that can be used. Colgate for children and Oral B toothpastes may be used if they are not mint-flavored. Patients can dip their toothbrushes in baking soda for the whitening and freshening benefits it provides. Acne soaps and preparations, dandruff shampoos, and corn removal products quite regularly include salicylic acid. It is also used to treat psoriasis and seborrheic dermatitis of the face and scalp, as well as to remove calluses. Plantar warts and common warts are attacked with various strengths of salicylic acid. It is prepared and sold as a gel, cream, lotion, or ointment. Acne is sometimes treated with a topical solution of straight salicylic acid. Some names, such as Sal-Clens shampoo and Hydrisalic, are dead giveaways, but other names, such as Clear Away or Freezone, provide no such clues that they contain salicylates.

Common Medications Containing Synthetic Salicylates

Alka Seltzer
Anacin
Asacol
Ascriptin (buffered aspirin)
Aspergum
Aspirin (acetylsalicylic acid)
Bayer Arthritis Pain Formula
Bengay
Bufferin
Darvon Compound
Disalcid
Doan's Pills
Ecotrin
Empirin Compound
Excedrin (all except the one labeled "Aspirin-free")
Fiorinal
Halfprin
Lortab ASA
Monogesic
Myoflex
Pepto-Bismol
Percodan
Soma Compound
Trilisate
Zorprin

Common Topical Products Containing Synthetic Salicylates

Almay Fragrance-Free SPF 15 Oil Free Lotion
Buf-Puf Acne Cleansing Bar with Vitamin E
Clearasil Double Textured Pads Maximum Strength (and other products)
Compound W Gel/Liquid
Coppertone Shade Sunblock Stick SPF 30 (2-ethylhexyl salicylate)
Fostex Regular Strength Medicated Cleansing Bar (and other products)
Freshburst Listerine (methyl salicylate)
Listerex Golden Scrub Lotion (and other products)

Many adult toothpastes (Crest, Mentadent, Pepsodent, Aquafresh, Aim, etc.)
Night Cast Regular Formula Mask Lotion
Noxzema Anti-Acne Gel and Pads
Oxy Clean Medicated Cleanser (and other products)
Pernox Lotion Lathering Scrub Cleanser (and other products)
Propa pH Acne Cream Maximum Strength (and other products)
Stridex Super Scrub Pads (and other products)
Wart-Off Topical Solution

Salicylates and Cosmetics

Many women taking guaifenesin lament the loss of their cosmetics. Their chief complaint is that they must do without "natural" products. It seems impossible for them to give up items like jojoba oil face masks, almond oil skin creams, and cleansers with aloe and arnica. They insist at first that they are natural, more so than mineral oil, silica, and talc, when actually all of these substances are found in nature. It seems somehow more natural to them to put grapeseed oil from a plant on their skin than lanolin, which is obtained from another mammal, a lamb. It offers some of them little solace to learn that natural, nonplant products may be used without adverse effects.

We suggest a rethinking process for those considering guaifenesin. The FDA does not regulate the use of words such as "pure" and "natural" and cosmetic companies have no obligation to prove their claims. "Natural" on a label can apply to something that is part synthetic or a natural ingredient that was synthetically removed from the plant by a wholly unnatural process using some very potent man-made chemicals.

Whenever plants are added to cosmetics, preservatives must be added as well to maintain freshness, and all of these are chemicals, some of which are potent allergens and topical irritants.

The fact that the cosmetic companies are suddenly shoveling plant material into ordinary moisturizers and makeup is only a marketing tool. Very few plants have been shown to have any benefit to the skin, and few of us—even ecologically minded consumers—have stopped to think about the morality of plundering the earth's rainforests for unproven beauty claims. More than a few of our patients have actually been astonished when they stop using so many compounds at how much better their skin is. This may be simply because some of the plants in topical products are irritating to the skin, forcing the use of yet another product to soothe it. Many plants, such as allspice, citrus, clover, and peppermint are among those known to cause irritation and increase the sun-sensitivity of the skin. Among the soothing ingredients we rely on are mineral oil, glycerin, cyclomethicone, dimethicone, petrolatum, and polyethylene glycol, all of which are made in laboratories and are the mainstays of every skin cream before plant extracts are added to make them more marketable.

Should we avoid laundry detergents with phosphates?

Phosphates in detergents are no problem. The amount of phosphate utilized by the human body is so massive that avoiding it has little or no effect. Guaifenesin seems able to overcome the amounts we are exposed to in our diets and topical preparations.

The fact that something comes from a plant does not make it beneficial or even desirable. Natural poisons will kill just as effectively as synthetic ones. Tobacco comes from a plant; poison ivy, poison oak, hemlock, oleander, and toadstools are all well-known, potentially lethal toxins. Just think of how many people have hay fever, and you will start to appreciate the threat posed by a host of natural ingredients that can become quite unfriendly. Our bodies are not flowerbeds and nature did not intend for us to lather on or indiscriminately ingest everything in sight. More than one of our ancient ancestors must have gripped his abdomen in his death throes induced by some herb, berry, or plant. We have learned to avoid such things but pay little heed to what may still be a lesser toxin due to our own, peculiar sensitivities.

A book by Paula Begoun is especially useful in the search for good beauty products. *Don't Go to the Cosmetics Counter without Me,* first published in 1991, is updated regularly, and Ms. Begoun publishes a newsletter and has a Web site. You will find this information in the Resources section of this book. Her book reviews literally thousands of products from companies such as Almay, Avon, the Body Shop, Charles of the Ritz, Dior, Coty, Revlon, Estée Lauder, Maybelline, and Vaseline Intensive Care. We are constantly reminded that results are what matter, and price and exotic ingredients do not necessarily guarantee a better product. Although the book does not list ingredients for each product, it gives a general overview of ingredients in cosmetics. The Appendix of Ms. Begoun's book provides toll-free numbers for cosmetic companies, a wonderful resource if you have questions about specific products and have a habit of throwing away packaging.

In her book, Ms. Begoun also evaluates cosmetic ingredients, both natural and synthetic, for their effectiveness. She gives her readers an inside look at the way cosmetics are created, manufactured, and marketed that is especially interesting and helpful to patients using guaifenesin. This book includes information on glycerin, animal and mineral oils as well as the minerals themselves, all of which contain no salicylates, are natural, and have proven benefits to the skin.

Recently, Andrea Rose, one of my patients, started a salicylate-free product line, *Andrea Rose Salicylate Free Skin Care* (contact information is included in the Resources section). Andrea has suffered from fibromyalgia for many years and has used guaifenesin since July 1996. Like many women, Andrea says that her most challenging task was to find salicylate-free skin care products and cosmetics. Out of this frustration her company was born. She has vowed that her products will forever remain guaifenesin-friendly. Andrea Rose products have many loyal users, one of whom explains: "It feels so good not to have to worry about whether or not something has salicylates in it."

Although it certainly seems complicated at first, it soon becomes routine to check cosmetic labels for offending ingredients. Lipsticks made with castor or camphor oil cannot be used, but many are made with lanolin or mineral oils. Face creams with beta-hydroxy cannot be used, but alpha-hydroxy preparations are acceptable. Lac-Hydrin, a potent synthetic alpha-hydroxy, is available by prescription for very dry skin. Retin-A and Renova will not block guaifenesin. Mascaras which do not touch the skin are no problem, just as nail polishes cannot block. Hair conditioners with natural balsam must be replaced with synthetic balsam, glycerin, panthenol, and the like. New scientific evidence suggests that sunscreens made from titanium dioxide are far more effective in reducing the effects of the sun than are the salicylate formulas. Toners with witch hazel must be traded for toners without it, and there is even a wide selection of acne products without salicylic acid, which has proven too irritating for some skin.

> *I have eliminated all salicylates from my topically applied products and still don't notice any effect from the guaifenesin. What should I do now?*
>
> Recheck everything, even your chewing gum and breath mints for natural mint flavorings such as peppermint, spearmint, or wintergreen. Search your vitamins and supplements for bioflavonoids, rose hips, or other botanical additions. If you still find no indication of salicylates ask your doctor to raise your dosage of guaifenesin.

It is possible to find good, high-quality products in all price ranges for all skin types while still avoiding salicylates. Our women's army of patients, armed with cosmetic dictionaries and the desire to get well, has proven this fact over and over again.

🐚 CONCLUSION

How do I sum up such an involved chapter? It seems to me I have repeated only one theme. *Get as far away as possible from anything that might even remotely contain salicylates.* I hope that all guaifenesin users will be as aware as we are of the depressing thought that something lurking in so many places can so completely block their road back from fibromyalgia. Yes, I am sorry that you will have to become your own expert. There is no shortcut. My earlier patients were the inadvertent laboratories that introduced us to the mutual hunt-and-peck system that finally produced this chapter. It is the story of their success I am recounting.

> *I'm finally having some good days again. I discovered that a vitamin with bioflavonoids from natural sources, including vitamin C from rose hips, was blocking the guaifenesin.*
>
> Last week, I drove four and a half hours to help my daughter, who was ill. It took a lot of energy to care for her baby and her busy two-year-old, cook, grocery shop, and do laundry. I was amazed at how much energy I had and how little I ached. I could not have done that three months ago.
>
> —Mary Ellen Stolle, Network leader for the Vulvar Pain Foundation

This chapter will do a great deal to help you avoid the damned compound that it has become for all of us. When you begin thinking this is too difficult for you to perfect, think how badly you are feeling. If you want to experience the euphoria many of us have experienced, let yourself get well for even one day and these will seem like small sacrifices indeed.

Chapter 5

❧

Hypoglycemia, Fibroglycemia, and Carbohydrate Intolerance

The doctor determined that I was hypoglycemic . . . and he also explained that hypoglycemia and fibromyalgia often go hand in hand. There was a name for what I had, an actual medical term! And there were also Web sites with information I could read. I was less than thrilled when he told me about the diet I would be on . . . Sugar was a no-no, as was caffeine. . . . I gulped as he rattled off the list of the carbohydrates I should avoid, including the "Big Five" that figured heavily in my diet: pasta (my Italian heart literally broke in two) rice, potatoes, bananas, and corn. . . . The doctor handed me a list of the permissible and said "Good luck."

This diagnosis meant that a morning might come when I could open my eyes and actually feel good to be alive, without fear of pain. Now four months later, I am pleased to say that I've experienced many such mornings. . . . I have more energy, I sleep better, I'm in a better mood. Friends, family members and coworkers all say they've seen a change in me. . . . Six months ago I would not have thought such a change was possible. But thanks to my own stubbornness . . . and the dedication of my current doctor, I have finally found relief. I guess what my doctor and I have in common is that we refused to give up the search for answers and we chose to ignore people who said there were none. For us both, perseverance has definitely paid off.

—*Michelle Fisher, from a published article in*
Palos Verdes Peninsula News

🐚 HYPOGLYCEMIA AND CARBOHYDRATE INTOLERANCE

In 1964, I was treating a podiatrist who suffered from fibro-myalgia. Luckily for me, she had many scientific interests and she studied a great deal. During one of her checkups, she brought me a pamphlet describing hypoglycemia. As an endocrinologist, I was certainly familiar with severe hypo-glycemia, the kind where patients pass out on the floor seemingly without provocation or from an excessive amount of insulin taken by a diabetic.

> *Hypoglycemia*—From the Greek "hypo," meaning low, sugar (glyc) in the blood (emia). The accepted medical criterion for this condition is a blood sugar reading falling below 50 milligrams per deciliter.

As I studied the broad array of symptoms listed in the tiny booklet, I realized that if the descriptions were even fifty-percent accurate, I had been missing the chance to help a lot of sick people. The symptom list included: fatigue, irritability, nervousness, depression, insomnia, impaired memory and concentration, anxieties, dizziness, blurred vision, leg cramps, sugar craving, flushing, sweating, palpitations, and even diar-rhea. These are the *chronic* symptoms, as we now label them, as opposed to the more dramatic ones, which are the *acute* symptoms of hypoglycemia.

My podiatrist-patient had added unwittingly to my bur-

den since I was still in the process of understanding and defining the as-yet nameless disease, fibromyalgia. As I learned more
about hypoglycemia, the overlap in symptoms was tremendous
and quite confusing to me. Although I had been largely successful in treating fibromyalgic patients with gout medications
for about five years, there were still a significant number of
them that remained partially ill. I could palpate a very obvious
improvement in their lumps and bumps, and they did complain less of their former pains. Since these findings and most
of their other symptoms were disappearing, these patients
should have been experiencing some perfectly normal days.
But that was not the case; in spite of the fact that they had less
pain and felt somewhat better overall, they were still miserable.

It was a bit startling to realize how many of my fibromyalgic patients also had hypoglycemia. Luckily, the treatment for
hypoglycemia was well known and highly effective. No medication is necessary or even useful. Treatment simply requires
eating the proper diet. The dilemma we had faced with our
partially responsive fibromyalgic patients was suddenly clari-
fied. Once both fibromyalgia and hypoglycemia were controlled, our patients recovered. It was wonderfully reassuring
that neither of these illnesses could leave any permanent damage. With adherence to the diet now added to their medication
for fibromyalgia, this last group of patients could be restored
to normal health with no traces of what had been labeled, in
our ignorance and frustration, hypochondriasis.

Finally, it was clear that two totally remediable diseases ac-
counted for all of their multiple complaints. As I gained experience, it became progressively easier for me to separate the two
conditions and treat both at the same time, and I was no
longer confused by patients with incomplete responses.

I had just begun to hope that I would finally be able to live without the pain from fibromyalgia. The guaifenesin treatment from Dr. St. Amand gave back my energy and mobility. It was all the more difficult, then, to be disabled by headaches.

I was aware that my health was not good, so I ate a vegetarian diet and followed the food pyramid recommendations closely; I ate a diet rich in carbohydrates and low in fat, and the worse I felt, the more carefully I followed these recommendations. Despite this, I was always hungry and faint, and my headaches were steadily worsening.

Claudia showed me the diet recommended for hypoglycemia and offered me the hope that by following this regimen I could control my headaches. I would have tried anything; I had nothing to lose. In fact, I had a lot to lose: pain, fatigue, and even excess weight. From one day to the next my headaches all but vanished; during the first few weeks my migraines diminished to one or two a week and I had no other headaches, either mild or severe. The improvement was so immediate and so unmistakable that I had no difficulty whatsoever following the diet, even though it was just before Christmas and I was surrounded by sweets.

—*Cynthia C., East Lansing, MI*

My education and enlightenment progressed, and I became more familiar with patients who had hypoglycemia as a stand-alone illness as well as those who suffered from simultaneous fibromyalgia. At the time, I was a spokesman for the Los

Angeles County Medical Association. *NBC News* wanted to present a segment on hypoglycemia, which was fast becoming the new fad of medicine. Because I was an endocrinologist, I was interviewed and had to discuss the condition on camera. I was featured along with physicians I had recommended who were full-time endocrinology staff members from two UCLA campuses. The story was shown on three consecutive evenings as five-minute, serialized segments during the prime-time newscast. Then, due to overwhelming viewer response, the program was shown a few more times in the following months. The Los Angeles County Medical Association, UCLA, and Harbor General Hospital were bombarded with phone calls. Since I was the only physician interviewed who was in private practice, all of the inquiries were referred to my office. I was inundated with calls requesting appointments from hypoglycemics, fibromyalgics, and combinations of the two, as well as from patients who were ill with many other conditions. Many of those I saw had been misdiagnosed, just as I would have done only a few years earlier. My patient base grew rapidly to include people not only from our county, but also from adjacent counties and other parts of California. Their sheer numbers provided me with a huge amount of information and instruction.

Carbohydrates—Chemicals made up of carbon, hydrogen, and oxygen which provide the body with one of its two main sources of energy along with fats. Sugars and starches are carbohydrates. Although we usually read about two types of carbohydrates, simple and complex, there are actually three classifications: mono-saccharides (glucose, galactose, fructose), disaccharides (sucrose, lactose, maltose), and polysaccharides (starch, cellulose). Ingested carbohydrates raise the blood sugar, and the pancreas responds with the release of insulin.

Simple carbohydrates—Sugars including table sugar (sucrose), fruit sugar (fructose), honey (maltose), and milk sugar (lactose).

Complex carbohydrates—Starches such as bread, pasta, rice, potatoes, cereals, peas, and beans.

To understand hypoglycemia better, we should first review the body chemistry that follows when one eats a carbohydrate such as a candy bar, a serving of potato, pasta, or rice. All these foods stimulate the release of insulin, a hormone with widespread functions. Nature, as usual, is skillfully adapted to conserve and maximize food storage. It designed our bodies to be frugal of its nutritive finds and to allow little waste. Ancient man did not often find food in overabundance. In fact, he might go a day or two without any nutrition at all. When he found sustenance, he devoured it on the spot. Rarely were all of the calories in this delightful repast needed for immediate use. Storage capabilities were necessary to provide energy on the less bountiful days that were sure to follow. Lean days would far outnumber his days of plenty. In modern times, our storage facilities are kept near overflow because calories are readily available. Every meal provides an excess caloric intake beyond our immediate needs.

Insulin—A hormone produced by the islets of the pancreas. Released in whatever amounts are needed to clear excess glucose from the bloodstream. Promotes the absorption of glucose into the liver and muscles, where it is stored as glycogen. Facilitates storage of amino acids and fats, known, therefore, as "the storage hormone." Without insulin, a person cannot gain weight.

Insulin, the only hormone that can direct excess calories (energy) into storage, is released promptly when carbohydrates are eaten, and attends to the work of conservation even before the meal is completed. Insulin is an insurance hormone that saves the surplus calories from each meal for future energy needs. It directs cells to store not only glucose, but also amino acids, the building blocks of protein, and fat. Insulin sends these stores to the body's largest energy warehouses, the muscle and fat cells. The liver also responds to insulin prodding, and initiates important metabolic effects. In the process of digestion, carbohydrates are completely converted to simple sugars and eventually to glucose. These sugars are delivered mainly to the liver and muscles, where insulin directs glucose storage in the form of glycogen. When this has been accomplished to maximum capacity, the remaining glucose is converted into fatty acids. These are hooked onto something called glycerol, and the combination is what we recognize as our body fat, or triglycerides. The liver packages these miniscule fat droplets for transport to all tissues, but they are directed mainly to the fat cells' storage depots. It is these droplets that make up the loathsome fat accumulations so many of us try to shed in the hope of restoring our normal body contour. Fat is nothing more than surplus energy maintained in the form of triglycerides. Our mouths and insulin—the caveman's lifesaving friends—are, in today's world of abundance, the enemies that help make us fat and ensure we stay that way.

Triglyceride—One of three "blood fats" that are known as lipids. It is the principal constituent of body fat. It is manufactured in the liver largely from the sugar and starches that you eat.

In certain people, the body is unable to process carbohydrates without adverse consequences. Hypoglycemia, or low blood sugar, is the name often used to denote a whole disease. But more accurately, it is only one of a cluster of symptoms that together make up a syndrome. Since it is actually far more than just low blood sugar, it could benefit from a better name. Patients with this condition actually suffer from a variety of insulin-related disturbances that are touched off by eating certain carbohydrates. (See figure 5.1.)

There are two ways to produce low blood sugar. It can be done by an excessive release of insulin. It can also be induced by a delayed or inadequate release of the hormones that are supposed to put the brake on the falling blood glucose. These are called the counterregulatory hormones because they counteract the effects of the insulin that is responsible for falling blood sugar. There are four of them, but adrenaline (epineph-

HYPOGLYCEMIA

Chronic Symptoms

- Fatigue, insomnia
- Nervousness, depression, irritability
- Dizziness, faintness
- Blurring of vision
- Ringing ears
- Gas, abdominal cramps, diarrhea
- Numbness/tingling of hands, feet, face
- Flushing/sweating
- Foot/leg cramps
- Bi-temporal or frontal headaches
- Impaired memory and concentration

Acute Symptoms

- Heart pounding
- Palpitations or heart irregularities
- Panic attacks
- Nightmares and severe sleep disturbances
- Faintness or syncope
- Acute anxiety
- Hand or inner shaking/tremor
- Sweating
- Frontal headache or pressure

Figure 5.1

rine) is the most important one in the realm of our discussion. All kinds of abnormal possibilities exist because a little too much of this or too little of that creates a whole spectrum of effects. Any of the many defective combinations can cause trouble. If either insulin or adrenaline is released in inadequate or excessive amounts, the other one must decrease or increase its output to avoid hypoglycemia. They dance together, but at opposite ends of the ballroom.

Insulin drives blood sugar down, and adrenaline pushes it up, and they are supposed to work in harmony. In hypoglycemia, the adrenal gland releases adrenaline, but the customary fine adjustments are lacking. One or the other hormone gains the upper hand at different moments, and what should be a harmonious dance lacks synchrony. The pancreas acts first and fast by releasing insulin, which causes the excessive drop in the blood sugar that we call hypoglycemia. The adrenal gland, slow in its counterpoint, suddenly wakes up as if hit by a two-by-four and squirts out an excessive amount of adrenaline, causing the acute and very alarming symptoms. (See figure 5.2.) During the premenstrual week, estrogen and progesterone add greatly to this hormonal disharmony.

Hypoglycemia's acute symptoms are truly frightening. They occur usually three or four hours after eating a high-carbohydrate meal, and generally last from twenty to forty minutes. When especially intense, they are referred to as panic attacks caused by the *repetitive* releases of insulin that eventually provoke the other glands of the endocrine system into overactivity. As we have seen, adrenaline is the system's ultimate weapon. It is the fail-safe hormone that always stops the free fall in blood sugar, even if it is sometimes a bit late in re-

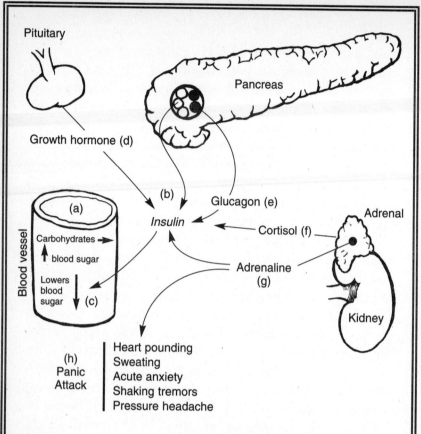

Pituitary

Pancreas

Growth hormone (d)

(b)

(a)

Insulin

Glucagon (e)

Adrenal

Cortisol (f)

Blood vessel

Carbohydrates →

↑ blood sugar

Adrenaline (g)

Lowers blood sugar ↓ (c)

Kidney

(h)
Panic
Attack

Heart pounding
Sweating
Acute anxiety
Shaking tremors
Pressure headache

Normal	Abormal
(a) Eating carbohyrates raises blood sugar.	Insulin lowers blood sugar too much; the brain reads "hypoglycemia" and stimulates release of:
(b) Bloodstream delivers sugar to the pancreas and releases insulin.	(d) growth hormone
	(e) glucagon
(c) Insulin enters bloodstream and lowers the blood sugar.	(f) cortisol
	(g) When these hormones cannot control insulin, the adrenal gland releases adrenaline, which stops insulin action within one to two minutes.
	(h) Adrenaline penalizes the body and causes acute symptoms.

Figure 5.2

sponding. Unfortunately, this is a good news, bad news situation, since it is adrenaline that is responsible for panic attacks. The symptoms of adrenaline release are quite familiar to everyone. We have all suffered from a sudden fright which causes the body to secrete this hormone. The results are heart pounding or irregularities and a feeling of severe anxiety. Shaking, hand tremors, drenching sweats, and frontal pressure headaches complete the picture. When these symptoms occur during the night, they are often preceded by nightmares. Sleep disturbances provoke daytime drowsiness and add greatly to the general fatigue.

Adrenaline (epinephrine)—A hormone released by the adrenal glands when the body senses imminent danger. It is sometimes called the "fight or flight hormone." It is designed to increase energy levels in emergencies. When the blood sugar falls in hypoglycemia, the body senses an emergency and releases adrenaline. This release normalizes the blood sugar within one to two minutes.

Endocrine system—Made up of glands that produce hormones (chemicals necessary to regulate the body's functions). They regulate or stimulate metabolism, growth, sexual development and function, and maintain the body in a state of balance (known as homeostasis).

So now you can understand my level of confusion when I realized I was now facing two conditions, often interlocked, for which none of my medical training had prepared me. I was forced to treat one condition, that was not well defined or understood, along with another that, in the eyes of my medical profession, might not even exist. This troubled me somewhat, since I did not enjoy veering away from well-accepted, well-researched medical treatments.

All of a sudden I was encountering far too many situations that I had not been taught how to handle. I had no choice but to look somewhere other than the bible of accepted medicine for successful treatments. It is spine-tingling in any field of work to walk over the threshold of uncertainty and come face to face with something exciting but entirely new. It was a little intimidating to find that a nameless disease was actually common, and equally astounding to realize that an existing medication could resolve the condition. I had been taught that results are what count. I remember one of my teachers during grand rounds who said emphatically: "Don't just stand there— do *something*!" I think this was his interpretation of the Hippocratic Oath, which could be paraphrased as: "get the patient well the best you can, but above all, do no harm." Treatment seemed simple, safe, and straightforward. I would recommend a diet to wipe out hypoglycemia, prescribe a medication for fibromyalgia, and enjoy the smugness that comes with success.

Making the Diagnosis of Hypoglycemia

The glucose tolerance test [is] . . . the worst torture in
a lab that can be done to anyone, especially a hypo-

glycemic. You arrive following a twelve-hour fast and then, while you are half-asleep, a needle is stuck into your arm and blood is drawn. Then you are given a drink called a GLU-Cola, which is basically a cola with half a bottle of Karo syrup poured into it. You have to drink this down fairly quickly without gagging, and then in an hour another needle is stuck in your arm, and blood is drawn again. They do this ten times during the next five hours. In between needle sticks you sit in a chair in a freezing sterile lab . . . and you can't walk around because it will cause you to release adrenaline and lower your blood sugar. And you can't eat anything, and you haven't eaten in seventeen hours by the end of the test. Somewhere around the fourth hour you feel like you are going to die, dizzy, sweating, sick, and then you feel like you are going to pass out. Just when you fall asleep, they wake you up to stick you again. When you finally get home you are horribly sick, and you stay dull-witted and dazed for several days.

—*C.C., La Jolla, CA*

The standard tool for making the diagnosis of hypoglycemia is the five-hour glucose tolerance test. A measured amount of glucose is administered to the patient, and if, during the course of the test, the blood sugar measurement falls below the magic number of 50 milligrams per deciliter (mg/dl), the diagnosis is confirmed. In my earlier days, we administered this test to every patient who admitted to any of the symptoms of hypoglycemia. To our surprise, many patients displayed normal sugar levels throughout the test. Despite this, they complained bitterly about a flock of hypoglycemic symptoms during their ordeal. We retaliated by drawing blood more often—every half-hour—hoping that more specimens would catch at least one low reading to prove our diagnosis correct. We soon noticed that the patient's symptoms were not necessarily synchronous with the timing of a blood sampling. It was already known in those days that, when the blood sugar falls sufficiently, the adrenaline release immediately counters insulin and reverses hypoglycemia. Since this occurs within one to two minutes, it made sense that, by the time a technician could insert a needle and draw a blood sample, glucose levels could have already returned to normal. We soon realized that our sampling was far too often missing the lowest blood sugar levels, so rapid was the adrenaline correction.

Finally, because our glucose testing failed to confirm our diagnosis fifty percent of the time, we decided to try a different approach to testing. We had our patients drink the same measured amount of glucose. This time, though, we omitted the blood sampling. Instead, our subjects simply recorded their symptoms during the next five hours in a little diary. We found that patients experienced all of the classic, acute symptoms of hypoglycemia. But I was also aware that these were the very symptoms that had made me suspect the diagnosis of hypoglycemia in the first place, before patients had been subjected to the ordeal of this five-hour test. I asked myself, if these patients are exhibiting the same symptoms without glucose, then why make them drink it at all? Were they not experiencing the same symptoms that diabetics develop in response to an insulin overdose? Why not just skip the test, take the patient's history, and accept the symptoms themselves as diagnostic for hypoglycemia?

I decided to use the test only if patients were suffering fainting spells or had an abnormally low *fasting* blood sugar. Either of those two factors prompted me to consider the possibility of an insulin-producing pancreatic tumor. This diagnostic approach worked even better. It saved patients five hours of testing, multiple needle sticks, a miserable morning, and the sick days that were sure to follow our sugar cocktail. After all, do you really need a blood sugar reading of below 50 mg/dl to tell you what you already know—that eating a lot of sugar or starch makes you feel lousy?

In 1994 Doctors Genter and Ipp published some interesting findings.[18] They performed a simple, elegant experiment that explained another reason why some patients with symptoms do not register the mandatory drop of blood sugar below 50 mg/dl. These two doctors ordered five-hour glucose tolerance tests on twenty young, healthy subjects who had no symptoms whatsoever of hypoglycemia. A catheter was placed in a vein so that blood could be sampled every ten minutes without repeated needle sticks. These samples were measured for the amounts of various hormones and the timing of their release as they played out their roles following the ingestion of a sugar load.

Surprisingly, about one-half of the subjects developed varying degrees of the acute symptoms, such as tremors, sweating, heart pounding, anxiety, or pressure headaches, during the test. Some had only a few of these effects, but others had all of them. As expected, the blood tests identified adrenaline release as the cause of these sensations. Very strangely, however, responses were induced with sugar levels quite in the normal range. The lowest was at 58 mg/dl of blood, but most had levels in the sixties, seventies, and one even in the eighties! This flew in the face of the accepted definition of hypoglycemia, that is, a blood sugar level below 50. This study and a later corroborating paper from France strongly suggest, at least to me, that we each have a set point for blood sugar. As it drops below our own unique, predetermined level, our brain says, "you're getting into trouble," and promptly triggers the hormonal and nerve impulses that are required to save us from passing out.

Now we only rarely perform the gold-standard, five-hour glucose tolerance test, since it is so unreliable in detecting hypoglycemia. Often a normal test fools a physician into thinking his or her patient does not have a carbohydrate problem. When we use symptoms alone for the diagnosis, it does not matter to what number the blood sugar might have fallen during a test. The term "hypoglycemia" should remain reserved for patients whose blood sugar drops below 50 mg/dl. We should look for a more accurate term for the group we are describing. The simple designation "carbohydrate intolerance syndrome" wins our vote. Regardless of blood sugar levels or which name we use, all patients with this symptom complex respond equally well to the same dietary restrictions.

Once I had a better understanding of carbohydrate intolerance, I was much better able to grasp the overlapping symptoms of fibromyalgia. (See figure 5.3.) Unless you or your doctor can recognize the distinctive complaints that help separate the two diseases, the second diagnosis may not be made. Then both patient and physician will assume guaifenesin treatment has failed, because only a partial success is achieved by treating just one of the two entities. The two diseases share many symptoms: fatigue, irritability, nervousness, depression, insomnia, flushing, impaired memory and concentration. Anx-

Relationship of Fibromyalgia and Hypoglycemia

Fibromyalgia	Overlapping Symptoms	Hypoglycemia
Skipping heartbeats (palpitations)	Ringing in the ears	Hunger tremors
Headaches (a) generalized	Weakness	Pounding heart
(b) neck-occiput	Fatigue	Panic attacks
(c) half-head	Irritability	Faintness
Dizziness (a) imbalance	Moodiness	Fainting
(b) vertigo	Nervousness	
Eye irritation	Depression	
Salt craving	Insomnia	
Eye dryness	Impaired memory	
Abnormal tastes	Impaired concentration	
Restless legs	Anxiety	
Constipation (IBS)	Frontal headache	
Burning urination (dysuria)	Dizziness	
Bladder infections	Blurred vision	
Interstitial cystitis	Numbness (face or	
Brittle nails	extremities)	
Itching anywhere	Abdominal cramps	
Rashes (a) hives	Gas	
(b) eczema	Bloating	
(c) neurodermatitis	Diarrhea	
(d) itchy blisters	Sugar craving	
(e) acne	Sweating	
Growing pains	Weight gain	
Vulvodynia (vaginal pain or irritation)	Generalized muscle stiffness	
Sound sensitivity	Nasal congestion	
Pain (a) muscles	Leg/foot cramps	
(b) tendons		
(c) ligaments		
(d) joints		

Figure 5.3

ieties are also common to both conditions, as are frontal or bitemporal headaches, dizziness, faintness, and weakness. Each can produce blurred vision, nasal congestion, ringing in the ears (tinnitus), numbness, and tingling of the hands, feet, or face. In addition, excessive gas, abdominal cramps, loose stools, or diarrhea are frequent. Many complain of leg or foot cramps. When hypoglycemia is the cause of these chronic symptoms, they are experienced even in the presence of a normal blood sugar level. This is because of the extensive endocrine and metabolic imbalances brought about by months of insulin-induced stress. (Refer to the Technical Appendix to review the involvement of various endocrine glands.)

There is a certain stiffness of muscles in hypoglycemia, but it is not the same as the pains from the lumps and bumps of fibromyalgia. Simply using one's hands to map swollen areas makes it possible to separate the two illnesses with considerable accuracy. Yet overall, the acute symptoms of carbohydrate intolerance remain the more dependable ones for making the diagnosis, just as the presence of lumps and bumps easily identify fibromyalgia. This is important, because hypoglycemia without the presence of fibromyalgia requires no medication.

❧ THE HYPOGLYCEMIA TREATMENT PROPER DIET

Before I started the diet, I was weak and shaky every few hours. I started eating some nuts for a protein jolt between meals, and eating smaller meals. Having been on the diet for eleven months, I notice I no longer get hungry between meals. My appetite is not as big and I don't get the shakes when I get hungry (unless I don't eat eventually). I don't have headaches all the time now and I don't have the afternoon crash at 2 to 3 P.M. anymore. It really helps you feel better. . . . I will stick to this diet, because when I've cheated and eaten sugar, I get a headache and feel very sleepy for hours. If you're experiencing a lot of pain, give it a try.

—*Heather Lock, Texas*

Many people ask if they should eat more carbohydrates because they are hypoglycemic. The answer is an emphatic "No!" In fact, quite the opposite is true. It is not necessary for anyone to load their diet with carbohydrates, because the body can easily manufacture all it needs. Despite this fact, it is common for people to consume carbohydrates in the belief that they will be superenergized. Sugars and starches raise the blood sugar about five minutes after they have been consumed. Proteins, and to a lesser extent fats, also provide fuel for the liver to raise glucose levels, but this takes about fifteen to twenty minutes. The liver and kidneys can easily convert some amino acids into glucose. If patients are not adversely affected by eating carbohydrates, we salute their stalwart metabolism. On the other hand, if eating carbohydrates induces the symptoms we are discussing, then what choice remains but to give them up?

Hypoglycemia can only be controlled with a perfect diet, one that eliminates all of the dangerous carbohydrates. As stated above, it is not necessary to add any foods; rather, it is the foods that one removes that determine a satisfactory recovery. Patients must not eat table sugar, corn syrup, honey, sucrose, glucose, dextrose, or maltose. Lactose (milk sugar) and fructose (fruit sugar) can be consumed in limited amounts only. For example, a glass of juice contains more fructose than is allowed on our diet, because it takes several pieces of squeezed fruit to make a glassful. Only one piece of fruit should be eaten in a four-hour period. All heavy starches must be avoided, including potatoes, rice, and pasta. Caffeine intensifies and prolongs the action of insulin, and so it is also forbidden. Alcohol, also a carbohydrate, can be consumed only after the blood sugar has been stabilized, and then only in limited amounts.

The elimination of all sugars (simple carbohydrates) as well as heavy starches (complex carbohydrates) is mandatory because they cause the body to release so much insulin. If insulin is not released, hypoglycemia will not occur. It is that simple. In time, each of the affected endocrine glands recovers. In my experience, recovery begins with a display of somewhat more energy somewhere between the fifth and tenth day after starting the diet. Some patients feel more fatigue during the first few days as they change their basic energy fuels from carbohydrates to protein and fat. During this initial period, patients may also experience headaches from both caffeine and carbohydrate withdrawal. The energy surge that eventually begins may be delayed for those who have been ill for a very long time. Total elimination of sugar and starch may seem like a monumental challenge, but with diligence and willpower, patients can do it successfully.

> I have been able to cautiously—and occasionally incautiously—reintroduce a few carbohydrates into my life, learning what my tolerance level is. But I am not tempted to add many; I have my life back, and compared to that, sweets and starches are a truly insignificant sacrifice.
>
> —*Cynthia C., East Lansing, MI*

Below are the foods that must be completely eliminated from your diet to overcome and control hypoglycemia.

Forbidden Foods List for Hypoglycemics: Foods to Avoid Strictly

Sugar in any form, including soft drinks
Caffeine in any form, including soft drinks
Fruit juices and dried fruits
Baked beans
Black-eyed peas (cowpeas)
Garbanzo beans (chickpeas)
Refried beans
Lima beans
Lentils
Potatoes
Corn
Bananas
Barley
Rice
Pasta of any kind
Burritos (flour tortillas)
Tamales
Sweets of any kind
Dextrose, maltose, sucrose, glucose, fructose, honey, corn syrup, or
  starch

Our diet for hypoglycemia is divided into two parts: "strict" and "liberal." Both diets will control hypoglycemia equally well. The strict diet was devised for those patients who need to lose weight; the liberal diet is designed for weight maintenance. The list of Foods to Avoid Strictly, above, applies to both diets, and must not be ignored.

You can eat as much as you like of all foods on the list below except for one of the few items with a quantity limit next to it. You can eat whenever you are hungry—there is no added benefit from eating less. If you don't see it on this list, you can't have it. Always check packaged products carefully, reading the ingredient list to make sure none of the foods to avoid are listed.

Dr. St. Amand's Strict Diet for Hypoglycemia and Weight Reduction

Meats

All meats are allowed, except cold cuts that contain sugar. (Check labels carefully. Low-fat or nonfat and turkey cold cuts usually have dextrose or corn syrup added. Bacon and ham are acceptable although they do list sugar on the labels. This sugar, however, cooks off and is not a problem. Hams that are heavily coated should be washed free of sugar.)

All fowl and game, fish, and shellfish are allowed in unlimited quantities

Dairy Products

Eggs

Any natural cheese (natural cheese is any cheese you slice yourself)

Cream (heavy and sour)

Cottage and ricotta cheeses (1/2 cup limit)

Butter and margarine

Fruits
Fresh coconut
Avocado (limit 1/2 per day)
Cantaloupe (limit 1/4 per day)
Strawberries (limit 6–8 per day)
Lime or lemon juice (limit 2 tsp per day) for flavoring

Vegetables
Asparagus
Bean sprouts
Broccoli
Brussels sprouts
Cabbage (limit 1 cup per day)
Cauliflower
Celery
Chard
Chicory
Chinese cabbage (limit 2 cups per day)
Chives
Cucumber
Daikon (long, white radish)
Eggplant
Endive
Escarole
Greens (mustard, beet)
Jicama
Kale
Leeks
Lettuce
Mushrooms
Okra
Olives
Parsley
Peppers (red, green, yellow, etc.)
Pickles (dill, sour, limit one per day)
Pimiento
Radicchio
Radish
Rhubarb
Salad greens
Sauerkraut
Scallions (green onions)
Snow peas
Spinach
String beans (green or yellow)
Summer squash (crook neck yellow, green)
Tomatoes
Water chestnuts
Watercress
Zucchini

Nuts (limit 12 per day)

Almonds	Macadamia nuts
Brazil nuts	Pecans
Butternuts	Pistachios
Filberts	Sunflower seeds (small
Hazelnuts	handful)
Hickory	Walnuts

Desserts

Sugar-free Jell-O

Custard (made with cream and artificial sweetener)

Cheesecake (no-crust or nut crust with cream cheese, sour cream, and artificial sweeteners)

Beverages

Artificially sweetened drink mixes like Crystal Light, Country Time, etc.

Club soda, zero-carbohydrate flavored soda waters

Decaffeinated coffee

Sodas with no sugar or caffeine

Weak or decaffeinated tea

Caffeine-free diet sodas

Bourbon, cognac, gin, rum, scotch, vodka, dry wine (after a month or two on a perfect diet, most hypoglycemics can tolerate one drink)

Condiments and Spices

All spices including seeds (fresh or dried), all imitation flavorings, horseradish

Sugar-free sauces such as hollandaise, mayonnaise, mustard, ketchup, soy sauce, Worcestershire sauce

Sugar-free salad dressings

Oil and vinegar (all types)

Miscellaneous
All fats
Caviar

If cholesterol is a problem, avoid cold cuts except sugar-free turkey. Trim all visible fat off meat. Remove the skin from poultry. Broil or grill foods instead of frying. Avoid full-fat cheese, heavy cream, solid margarine, hollandaise sauce, and macadamia nuts. Use egg whites or Egg Beaters instead of whole eggs. Use liquid margarine only. Nuts should be dry roasted only. Use canola or olive oil.

Dr. St. Amand's Liberal Diet for Hypoglycemia and Weight Maintenance

(Add these foods to the strict diet)

Fruits (limit: one piece of fruit every four hours. No fruit juices)
Apples
Apricots
Blackberries (1/2 cup limit)
Blueberries (1/2 cup limit)
Boysenberries
Casaba melon (1 wedge limit)
Grapefruit
Honeydew melon (1 wedge limit)
Lemons
Limes
Nectarines
Oranges
Papaya
Peaches
Pears

Plums
Raspberries
Strawberries
Tangerines
Tomato juice
V-8 juice

Vegetables
Artichokes
Beets
Carrots
Onions
Peas
Pumpkin
Squash (winter such as acorn, butternut, fresh pumpkin, spaghetti, etc.)
Turnips

Nuts
Cashews
Peanuts
Soy Nuts

Dairy Products
Whole, nonfat, low-fat milk and buttermilk
Unsweetened Yogurt

Desserts
Sugarless diet puddings (1/2 cup a day limit)

Breads
Three slices a day of sugar-free white, whole wheat, sourdough, or light rye. No more than two slices at one time *or* 3 servings a day of sugar-free flat bread (no more than two servings at a time)

Miscellaneous
Carob powder
Flour, gluten or soy only
Gravy made with gluten or soy flour only
Wheat germ
Puffed rice, shredded wheat, or other sugar-free cereals
One-cup popcorn (popped)
2 tacos or 2 enchiladas (2 corn tortillas only)

Most of the questions we are asked about the diet arise out of confusion about the nature of carbohydrates themselves. Many people have difficulty understanding why they cannot eat a small amount of potato instead of the three slices of sugar-free bread a day that the diet allows. They are accustomed to diets in which calories are simply added up. On a caloric restriction diet, the total number of calories from meat, cake, or potato is simply added up, and if the total number is kept low enough, weight loss will continue without regard for the dietary mix. So carbohydrate substitution, gram for gram, seems logical. But this type of math does not work with carbohydrates since not all carbohydrates are created equal. They vary greatly in their ability to release insulin.

The Glycemic Index of Foods (GI) ranks foods on how they affect blood sugar levels in comparison to straight glucose. It is mainly used for evaluation of the metabolism of carbohydrates, since protein and fat do not cause the blood sugar to rise very much unless they are eaten together with those carbohydrates. Initially devised with glucose as 100, it is now more common in America to see white bread set as 100. (In our text we will use the original scale, with glucose as 100. To convert to the white-bread scale multiply by 0.7.)

Tables have been devised that make food comparisons by the amount blood sugar rises following their ingestion. These charts describe a "glycemic index" of foods. The base reference is usually sugar (glucose), which is assigned the number 100. A potato, which contains glucose molecules strung together, is 98. On the other hand, fruits contain fructose, which does not raise blood sugar to the same extent and releases far less insulin. A peach, for example, has a glycemic index of 26. Though both fructose and glucose are carbohydrates, you can readily see why one cannot substitute the grams of one for the other. Foods with a high glycemic index are excluded from the hypoglycemia diet, foods with a lower one can be consumed in moderation, and the lowest foods can be eaten in unlimited quantities.

When we first designed our diet, we had to rely on our patients as teachers and test subjects, because the glycemic index had not yet been invented. Any food that induced symptoms of hypoglycemia in even one of our patients was placed on the list of forbidden foods. This provided us the assurance that our diet would always resolve the symptoms of carbohydrate intolerance, and thirty years later, it still holds up.

Twenty Common Foods and Their Glycemic Index[19]			
Fructose	25	White bread	69
Yogurt	32	Brown rice	66
Milk	34	White rice	72
Tomatoes	38	Wheat bread	72
Apples	39	Cornflakes	80
Pasta	45–50	Honey	87
Peas	53	Carrots	92
Sucrose	59	Baked potato	98
Sweet corn	59	(russet)	
Corn	59	Glucose	100
Bananas	62		

When using other low-carbohydrate diet lists and recipes, the hypoglycemic patient must always be on the alert. Most low-carbohydrate diets were designed for weight loss alone, and will not always control hypoglycemia. One must always check ingredients and packaging to make sure that nothing slips in to destroy all of the benefits of the previous restrictions.

In our experience, about two months of perfect dieting are

needed to wipe out all the symptoms attributable to carbo-hydrate intolerance. Consider the entire dietary process as if one were building a checking account. First, deposits must be made. The hypoglycemia diet builds energy reserves to the highest amount attainable for each individual. When sufficient funds are available, patients can begin writing checks, but they must remember that the balance in their account drops each time one is written. When the account is full, one can begin experimenting with "dangerous" carbohydrates. Each carbohy-drate consumed is a debit, and depletes the account by a cer-tain amount. Patients cannot overspend without taking time out to replenish reserves, or their symptoms will return. And if hypoglycemics are not careful, their accounts will be totally wiped out again. At that point, the only solution is to brace for the adrenaline surges and panic attacks that follow. Then they must start over again, building up their reserves. It is much better to heed the early warning signals and return to the diet without deviation for a time. This is the key to damage control.

Patients should make a great effort to determine what their first symptom is after excessive dietary indiscretions. This is usually increased fatigue, or it may be a frontal, pressure-type headache. Gradually, hypoglycemics learn exactly what they can allow themselves. They will become aware that emotional or physical strain will make them more vulnerable, since stress places greater demands on their energy bank. The premen-strual period is also notoriously fragile. At these times it is more difficult to maintain an adequate reserve, which makes it far easier to slip into deficit spending. It is better to cut back on carbohydrates without waiting for multiple symptoms to force the issue.

No physician or dietitian can predict what dietary restrictions will ultimately be necessary. Hypoglycemics are often rewarded with greater dietary leeway when their fibromyalgia begins to clear. Once their tissues eliminate the excess phosphate, and proper energy production resumes, they lose some or all of their susceptibility to hypoglycemia. For others, the great individual variability among hypoglycemics means that their cheats will have to be well timed and well planned for years.

> I got on the liberal hypoglycemia diet and have dramatically improved since then. I feel clear-headed with very little muscle pain on most days. . . . If I cheat on my diet more than once or twice a week, I pay with nervousness, fatigue, and pain. I had serious withdrawal from refined carbohydrates. It felt like an addiction to me. I now look at foods as nourishment, not a reward or something to soothe me.
>
> —*Heather Lock, Texas*

FIBROMYALGIA + HYPOGLYCEMIA = FIBROGLYCEMIA

Our statistics show that about forty percent of women and twenty percent of male fibromyalgics have hypoglycemia or carbohydrate intolerance. (See figure 5.4.) Because it is a more accepted term, we use the name "hypoglycemia" in any patient who experiences the repetitive adrenaline-release symptoms. Most of our patients developed their symptoms sometime after the onset of fibromyalgia, so we wanted a name for patients who have both conditions—fibromyalgia and carbohydrate intolerance. We have chosen "fibroglycemia."

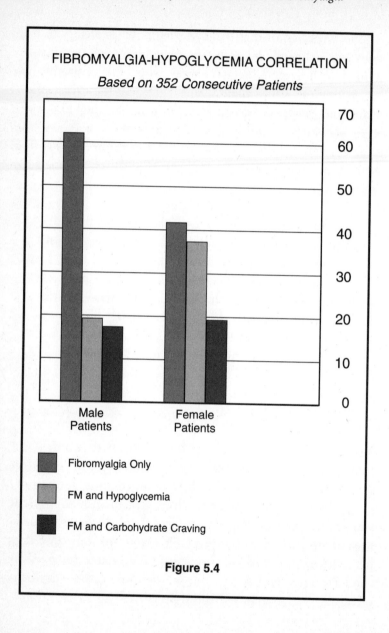

Figure 5.4

So what, you ask, is the reason that fibroglycemia is so common in our patients? We've already described the mapping system we use to make the diagnosis of fibromyalgia, and how our hands can easily identify the swollen areas of the body as contracted portions of muscles, ligaments, and tendons. These areas are swollen mainly because of accumulated intracellular fluid under high pressure. But they are also *working* tissues in their spastic, contracted state. Their constricted segments are pulling on bones, joints, or adjacent tissues twenty-four hours a day without relief. Such working structures quickly fatigue and begin to ache just as they would from a never-ending, low-grade workout. We are also aware that, for every lump and bump we put on the map, there are many other affected structures too deep for us to feel, and these are invisible accomplices in this metabolic frenzy that leads to exhaustion. Those who exercise stop exercising when it hurts, but fibromyalgics cannot stop their muscles from working.

Remember that the currency of energy for all cells is ATP. Eighty to ninety percent of our food is converted into this substance. Every bodily function demands huge supplies of this chemical. One cannot even think without using large amounts of ATP for brain activity. Ounce for ounce, the central nervous system—especially the brain—uses more than any other tissue. Fingernail and hair growth, digestion, fat deposition, breathing, urinating, fighting infections, or healing tissue trauma all utilize ATP. The bulk of ATP production and consumption, however, occurs through muscle activity. As overworked tissues fatigue, they use nerves to signal the need for more fuel. The brain receives the message, and the resulting thought is: "I'm tired. Give me a candy bar." When ATP production is normal, energy should be available within five minutes of eating most carbohydrates. This is not true for fibromyalgics. In these patients ATP formation is defective and no amount of eating will satisfy the demand for energy, especially because of the unrelenting work being done by their muscles.

Most fibromyalgics repetitively yield to their carbohydrate cravings throughout the day in a futile attempt to create energy. Since sugars and starches are quickly converted to glucose in the process of digestion, the body prefers them for fuel. Unfortunately, the carbohydrate-craving fibromyalgics quickly saturate their systems with glucose molecules that cause the pancreas to release large amounts of insulin. Insulin surges lower the blood sugar by driving it mainly into muscles, but also into fat cells, the liver, and most other areas of the body. These repeated insulin spurts will also eventually cause hypoglycemia in genetically susceptible individuals. The symptoms of hypoglycemia are then compounded with those of fibromyalgia, and the result is a miserable-feeling fibroglycemic.

These are the sickest of our patients. For them, dietary modification is not just a good idea, it is mandatory. They face a huge metabolic chore. They must eat themselves out of hypoglycemia while simultaneously accepting the increased symptoms of fibromyalgia reversal. There can be no compromise for this group, or they will continue to feel terrible even after the medication has purged much of the fibromyalgic debris from their tissues. Fibroglycemics must either choose to eat correctly or not feel any better.

Since being diagnosed with fibromyalgia and hypoglycemia, I've been experimenting with my carbohydrate intake, and I've been able to deduce that my hypoglycemia is pretty severe and is made a lot worse by the fibromyalgia. When I am in a bad fibromyalgia episode, I've found that it is critical that I do not deviate from the strict diet *at all*. Even one piece of bread can trigger a noticeable increase in all my symptoms. Also, there seems to be a very direct relationship between my carbohydrate intake and my depression. When I am very faithful to the strict diet, my depression quiets down. There have been short periods of time when I experienced real mental peace. If I botch the diet, the first casualty seems to be that sense of peace.

—*G.W., Los Angeles*

We have noticed that obesity offers some protection against hypoglycemia. This is actually unfortunate, because these chubby cells are provoking more serious disturbances. The fatter a cell gets, the more resistant it becomes to further storage attempts by insulin. It is much more difficult to prod obese cells into opening their transport tunnels when they consider themselves already fat enough. As a result, less amino acids (building blocks for protein) and fatty acids can be inserted into the usual sites. The pancreas, ever-mindful of the waste-not-want-not principle, presumes its message is not being received. Rather than waste the digested food residues, the pancreatic islets instead increase their output of insulin. This is like hitting deaf fat and muscle cells with a two-by-four. Suddenly they respond, and storage proceeds.

The step beyond simple insulin resistance (as this metabolic state is called) is Type II, or adult-onset, diabetes. Cells that are unresponsive to insulin do not absorb glucose as easily as they once did. At this point the blood sugar level does not drop as abruptly and eventually it does not drop at all. In this way obesity can correct hypoglycemia and make patients *think* they have outgrown their sugar problem. (See figure 5.5.) But there is a heavy price to pay down the line. The health ravages of insulin resistance are many, and those of diabetes are many times worse. This is not a topic we plan to discuss in this book. It is sufficient here to simply warn that neither low nor high blood sugar is healthy.

Many fibromyalgics merely crave sugar but have not become hypoglycemic. They suffer all of the aches, pains, and fatigue of the others but at least have not added the adrenaline symptoms of the fibroglycemics. Carbohydrate cravers may feel some of the same symptoms as those who are intolerant to glucose at various times. During adverse situations, they could be pushed into the fibroglycemic syndrome by a heavy sugar binge, excessive alcohol intake, or unusual emotional stress, especially for women during their premenstrual week. The final push into fibroglycemia could also be a serious infection, trauma of any kind, including surgery or heavy dental work. Cravers can feel generalized improvement by sticking to the low-carbohydrate diet for one or two months. They may get an energy spurt that will encourage them while waiting for the guaifenesin to begin reversing their fibromyalgia. Most patients will feel some benefit from the diet, even if they are not fibroglycemic or cravers. Some quick rewards include the lifting of "fibrofog" and avoiding drowsiness after meals. Following this diet is worth a two-week experiment. If no improvement is felt, the diet can be abandoned as long as the person is not actually carbohydrate-intolerant. Those who merely crave carbohydrates would eventually get well without dieting, once there is significant fibromyalgia reversal. I must

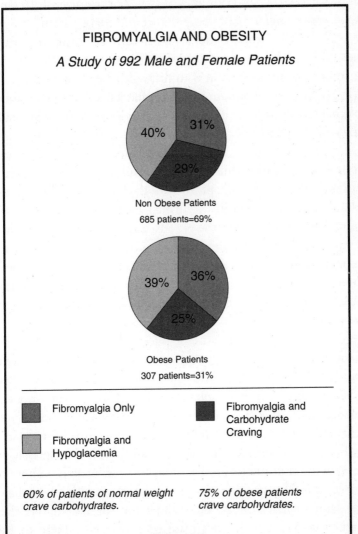

Figure 5.5

stress that *no specific diet is necessary for those who suffer only from fibromyalgia.*

There are other reasons, too, why less insulin release should help fibromyalgics as well as fibroglycemics. One of the prime functions of insulin is to drive glucose into cells, but always with a certain amount of phosphate, because one of phosphate's roles is to attach itself onto the glucose molecule inside the cell. In most structures of the body, this attachment prevents glucose from escaping from the interior stores and keeps it available for local energy needs. Insulin also signals certain kidney cells to reabsorb phosphate that was filtered from the blood for elimination in the urine. These phosphate ions are then delivered back into the bloodstream and transported back to many cells throughout the body. Some cells are especially responsive to the instructions of insulin and absorb considerable amounts of phosphate. Muscles are the most cooperative. The cells most severely affected in fibromyalgia are the very ones that respond best to insulin. My theory, you will recall, suggests that an excess amount of phosphate is what eventually slams the brakes on energy formation. The chemistry of fibromyalgia, hypoglycemia, and the combination disease, fibroglycemia, is certainly complex. In simple terms, if you have the wrong genes, and yield to your craving for carbohydrates, you will release more insulin and drive more phosphates into your cells. As this happens, you will certainly notice progressively less energy, and the rest of the symptoms will surely follow.

This is why, in our experience, fibroglycemia patients have the same beneficial response to the low-carbohydrate diet that hypoglycemics do. We urge fibroglycemics to adhere to the strict diet if they are overweight and to the liberal diet if they are not. Remember that both versions of the diet control blood sugar swings equally well. The only added benefit of the strict diet is weight loss, so patients who do not need to lose weight should avoid it.

> I stopped all my medications cold turkey and went on the hypoglycemia diet. I started guaifenesin and went through some bad cycles. I fell off my diet and suffered for that. But slowly things have gotten much better. I'm down twenty-five pounds in weight, my mind is clearing, my muscle spasms have cleared, and I can sleep. I am not perfectly well but I can make it through the day without having to lie down for most of it. The most important thing is that I now have a life.
> —*G.W., Los Angeles*

When treating fibroglycemics, we do not wait for the benefits of the diet before initiating the guaifenesin therapy. We simply have seen no reason for wasting time. When the hypoglycemia portion of the combined disease clears, usually with two months of a perfect diet, patients may begin adding carbohydrates and—just as in hypoglycemia—each individual must gradually define her own final limitations. And it is entirely possible that there will be no need for dietary restrictions once fibromyalgia stops its wanton destruction of energy.

I know of no modalities other than proper diet and the uricosuric medications that can reverse the mix of fibromyalgia and hypoglycemia. Discipline in avoiding salicylates and adherence to the proper diet are mandatory to restore well-being. There are few situations in medicine where success depends so greatly on the tandem efforts of patients and physician. It certainly falls upon the patient to help direct and control her or his recovery. It seems a lot to ask of a person who is already miserable—to give up favorite foods along with the many restrictions imposed by the need to avoid salicylates while taking guaifenesin. However, the appearance of the first good hours and days makes patients almost euphoric. The reward is great and highly exhilarating when contrasted with the preceding, disabling symptoms of these syndromes.

From the abyss of terrible to the heights of wonderful is not such a long climb. We have presented you, the patient, with a ladder. You will have to climb rung by rung or not only wallow where you are, but also continue your deeper descent into your personal hell. Those of us who have recovered are solicitous of your current status and urge you to join us in living.

❦ LIVING ON THE FIBROGLYCEMIA DIET

> Since I have begun treatment with guaifenesin for my fibromyalgia, my carbohydrate cravings have lessened and it is really not so hard to follow the hypoglycemia diet. I would have expected it otherwise—that with the worsening of symptoms, my carb cravings would have become intolerable. But that is not what I have experienced.
>
> —L.N., *Massachusetts*

First of all, take a deep breath. Once you are over the panic at the thought of giving up "everything" you eat, you will need to think about what you *can* eat. Most people start out slowly, hesitantly, and afraid to make a mistake. This is good, because, as we have said earlier in the chapter, dietary mistakes do have consequences for fibroglycemics. But after a month or two on the diet, nearly everyone gets creative.

The first meal of the day is breakfast, and breakfast is the meal we get the most questions about. Yet there are many choices! On the strict diet, eggs can be prepared any style, fried, boiled, or in omelets, with any of the usual additions—cheese, green pepper, sour cream, tomatoes, bacon, sausage, a small amount of avocado, and herbs. Any meat can be eaten, including bacon (even though it is sugar-cured, because frying it burns off all the sugar). Ham should be washed if the rind has been sugar-cured or honey-baked. Breakfast drinks can be made with protein powder (egg or soy), cream, and fruit or nut extracts. You can toss in strawberries if you do not need to save your quota for later in the day. You can have your scoop of cottage cheese with a slice of cantaloupe. Smoked salmon and cream cheese are quite acceptable, as are breakfast steaks and pork chops. We tend to think in terms of certain foods as being "breakfast foods." But really it is all the same to your digestive tract, so you can eat any of the acceptable foods in the morning. Egg custard made the night before with heavy cream, eggs, vanilla extract, and sugar substitute can be refreshing and delicious on a warm summer day. On the liberal diet you can add a piece of sugar-free toast with a bit of sugar-free peanut butter, or make a "smoothie" from fruit, tofu, milk, and sugar-free syrups. That should give you some breakfast ideas.

Lunch on the strict diet could include vegetables with or without meat. Deviled eggs make wonderful snacks as long as they are not stuffed with sweet relish and the mayonnaise is sugar-free. On the strict diet, of course, one has to improvise to make a sandwich. When I am on the strict diet, I use two cabbage leaves as my "bread." That way I have something to hold onto and to keep the meat or cheese in place! Salads with ground beef, chicken, cheese, sour cream, and avocado, or anything your imagination inspires, lend to the possibilities. You can have a salad—Caesar's, chef's, Cobb, egg, Greek, shrimp, tuna—as long as it contains no sugar, corn syrup, or honey in the dressing. The fast-food chains always make hamburgers or cheeseburgers available; just toss out the bun. Diagonal slices of daikon radish are great for adding cheese, pimiento, capers, or meats to serve as hors d'oeuvres. I am delighted that this is not a cookbook; I get hungry as I write! On the liberal diet one can have a serving of sugar-free bread or sugar-free flat bread with cream cheese, butter, sugar-free peanut butter, or sour cream.

Dinner on the strict diet usually conjures up bigger meals from the same ingredients that were used for lunch. We tend to prepare our chicken or meat somewhat differently—grilled or broiled instead of in salads or sandwiches. Fish is usually thought of as a dinner food, and can be fried, boiled, or baked. Meat and vegetables can be stir-fried together, roasted, baked, or grilled on the barbecue. Even on the strict list, there are many vegetables available. Use cauliflower, cubed daikon chunks, and even bits of squash instead of potatoes. Fry chicken with a batter made from egg and crushed pork rinds . . . delicious! Blackened chicken and fish are a dramatic change. Mushrooms can be stuffed with spinach and cheese. Stir-fry shrimp with bell peppers, mushrooms, or scallions, or scampi with extra butter and garlic. Grilling marinated vegetables such as eggplant, mushrooms, summer squash, and red peppers makes a nice variation. You can change basic recipes with the addition of spices such as white, green, or black pepper, paprika, curry powder, dried mustard, chili powders, and hot pepper sauces. Liquid smoke, horse-radish garlic paste, and Thai pepper sauces can be used on meat and vegetables. Best of all, if it's on the strict diet, you can have as much as you want. On the liberal diet, fake a pasta dish by using spaghetti squash with the usual sauces, or simply serve it with butter and Parmesan cheese. Celery root can be cooked and whipped into faux mashed potatoes! Artichokes with butter and sugar-free mayonnaise can be eaten as an appetizer, and don't forget that escargot and caviar can be eaten on both diets! Desserts that work for both diets are egg custards, sugar-free cheesecake, and Jell-O. We even have patients who make "ice-cream floats" with whipping cream added to diet root beer.

Eating out presents a major challenge to some fibro-glycemics. I have found that if one enlists the waiter's help, it's not terribly hard. Most restaurants will readily accommodate you and substitute vegetables in place of rice or potato. Cottage cheese or sliced tomatoes are another option. It is best to bring your own decaffinated coffee in a packet, as waiters sometimes mix up pots of coffee. You can order the same choices of meat or fish cooked as you would at home. Ask the waiter if their Caesar or blue-cheese dressings are sugar-free. If not, use oil and vinegar with or without a squeeze of lemon juice. Many restaurants now have delicious, flavored olive oils right on the table that can be put on salads or vegetables. In Mexican restaurants you can order fajitas, ropas viejas, or machaca; even the chili relleno is only lightly floured. Obviously, on the strict diet, do not eat the tortillas. Italian restaurants offer dishes like veal piccata or chicken, and often seafood such as scampi and calamari. The golden rule is to ask—and persevere until you find a choice (or a restaurant) that pleases you.

Substitutions for Adapting Nondiet Recipes to Ingredients for a Strict Low-Carbohydrate Diet

Sugar: Diabeticsweet, Sugar Twin, Stevia, Sucralose

1 tbsp. cornstarch: unflavored gelatin or 2 tbsps. gluten, soy flour or Atkins bake mix

Whole milk: 1 part cream to 1 part water (add a dash of sweetener because milk is sweeter than cream)

Buttermilk (one cup): 1/2 cup cream, 1/2 cup water, 1 tbsp. vinegar or lemon juice (let stand five minutes, tiny amount of sweetener—see above)

Fruit juice: fruit extract and sweetener to taste, Crystal Light Orange Juice, Lemonade

Bread crumbs: sunflower kernels crushed in a blender (unsalted), crushed pork rinds, or soy or egg protein powder

Flour for thickening: Atkins baking mix, soya flour, protein powder, egg protein powder, or water chestnuts mushed to a paste in a blender (you may have to add a little of their liquid)

Recently there has been a move towards lower-carbohydrate diets. This trend, along with the huge number of diabetics watching their sugar intake, has resulted in a boom of resources for those on our diet. Several excellent new cookbooks are available, and the Internet has a plethora of sites to help those on low-carbohydrate diets. Information on products is included along with recipes that can be downloaded for use on many occasions. Some of these are listed in the Resources section at the back of this book. Remember to check each and every recipe to make sure that ingredients not allowed on our diet are excluded. Sugar-free syrups, high-protein shakes with no carbohydrates, protein snack bars, protein powders, and sugar-free condiments are luckily no longer difficult to find.

It is not within the scope of this book to discuss fully the merits of fats versus carbohydrates as a source of fuel for the body. The battle has begun to rage in medicine, however. One fact stands out. Only one hormone can store fat in fat cells, and that is insulin. Insulin is released in response to carbohydrates, as we have already discussed. Fats do not release significant amounts of insulin, and proteins only a bit more *if they are not eaten with carbohydrates.* Protein and carbohydrates ingested together release much larger amounts than either one alone. Our strict diet permits weight reduction mainly because it avoids the release of insulin and because protein digestion and storage require more calories than are contained in the food itself.

For the purpose of this book, we will temporarily bow to the "party line" for a moment to suggest that one avoid *saturated* fats. (We are aware, however, that current reports show no reduction in heart deaths from past recommendations regarding fat abstinence.) Thus we urge the use of only unsaturated fats such as contained in vegetable oils and *liquid* margarines, and in moderation. We will continue to tell our patients that carbohydrates, both complex and simple, and sugars have been erroneously touted as beneficial, and society is just now beginning to face the consequences, including an explosion of obesity and adult-onset diabetes. Advocates including Drs. Robert Atkins, Michael and Mary Eades, and Richard Bernstein have made this point and have explained their positions eloquently.[20] For us it would require another whole book to explain our stance fully.

So let it suffice to say that we prefer to summarize as follows. We are *not* content with what has been preached. What has been promulgated in recent years is *not* healthy eating. The incidence of obesity is rising rapidly, as is its kin, diabetes. They both kill, as does a steady excess of insulin. Weight reduction *can* be achieved easily and comfortably with sufficiently low-carbohydrate intakes. Those who have tried to lose weight for years while eating the high-carbohydrate currently advocated would do well to give the low-carbohydrate diet a try. We understand the chemistry of foodstuffs but in no way will we attempt at this writing to superimpose our recommendations over those of personal physicians.

I have been on the low-carbohydrate diet for about thirty-three years. I am not hypoglycemic, but this diet has been a godsend, first to help me drop the few pounds I wanted to lose, and then to maintain my weight within a three-pound range. I confine myself to the strict diet during the week. That will normally drop my weight one or two pounds below my desired level and allow me to face the weekend in a more liberal mood. I confine my cheating at that time to eating pizza, rice, or bread. That is sufficient to keep me contented. Each of you will develop your own ritual of dieting and a cheating system. But first, you must get out of the hypoglycemia part of your fibroglycemia. In that process, why not take your weight down to a healthier level? After you have done this, allow yourself only enough cheats to ensure you smile every morning while standing on your scale.

Chapter 6

The Protocol

Last winter, I was ready to apply for Social Security disability payments. I only dared to drive my car one or two miles on a "good day." I hadn't had a social life for three years. My credit rating was ruined because I was so exhausted I would let bills pile up for months, then try to catch up with them all at once. . . . Nights were torture. I woke up every hour to hour and a half all night long. I had irritable bowel, irritable bladder, and restless legs. In the mornings, my joints ached so much that at times I was forced to get down on my hands and knees and crawl from the bedroom to the bathroom to the kitchen. . . .

By March, I'd decided I was willing to try guaifenesin. Maybe it wasn't for the faint of heart, but neither was the quality of the life I was living. . . . For the next several weeks I felt miserable most of the time and then, suddenly, I had two days of total reprieve from FMS. Not just "good" days—extraordinary, amazing days. Then I started into the next cycle. I've had all my old symptoms return in full force. . . . Tomorrow will be two months on guaifenesin and, according to the protocol, I should have reversed one year of symptoms of FMS by now. I can honestly say that I feel better than I did a year ago, and I certainly bounce back from exertion much faster than I used to. So, this isn't easy; it isn't fun; but it *works*. Follow the protocol to the absolute letter, be ruthless in getting rid of products and foods that aren't good for you, and go for it!

—*Anne*

It's time to take a closer look at our protocol itself, and lay each step out carefully. Understanding these steps and following them precisely are important. In this chapter we've tried to be as clear and concise as possible, without explanations of how and why. It's meant to be a road map to tell you exactly how to go about using guaifenesin to get well.

🐚 FIND A DOCTOR TO OBTAIN A DIAGNOSIS

The first thing to do is to make sure that you have fibromyalgia. This sounds obvious and even silly, but it is important. It's dangerous to treat yourself and to assume that all your symptoms are from fibromyalgia. If you have not yet been diagnosed, make an appointment with your doctor. When you make the appointment, be sure to mention that you suspect you have fibromyalgia. If the doctor you have called does not believe fibromyalgia exists or seems hesitant to treat it, don't make an appointment. Instead, call a different doctor. This may seem harsh, but because the road to recovery is a difficult one, you will want to have a doctor you can work with. It is too much to expect that a doctor who is not convinced fibromyalgia is real will turn out to be the partner you need.

If you need help finding a doctor, there are several things you can try. First of all, ask your friends. If one of them has a doctor he or she describes as a good listener or open-minded, this is a good place to start. You do not need a specialist to make the diagnosis of fibromyalgia. General practitioners or internists are perfectly qualified to help you. And because they are not specialists, they may have fewer preconceived notions.

Any physician or nurse practitioner able to prescribe medication in your state can treat you with guaifenesin.

Another possibility for finding a doctor is to call local fibromyalgia support groups. If there isn't an FMS group around, try the local chapter of the Arthritis Foundation. It usually has lists of doctors who are sympathetic to those with FMS. A hospital in your area may know of one. On-line newsgroups and Web sites may also have lists of doctors.

Once you are face to face with a doctor, what should you expect? If you have not had blood tests recently, the doctor will probably want to order them. A basic work-up will include a blood count to rule out anemia or infection because, like fibromyalgia, these can cause fatigue or muscle pain. You should also have a thyroid test known as a TSH. This sensitive test is the most accurate for checking thyroid function. An underactive thyroid can cause fatigue and other symptoms, so your doctor will want to make sure your gland is functioning normally. Thyroid conditions are not related to fibromyalgia, but they are more common in women than in men. Fasting blood sugar should be measured. High (diabetes) or low blood sugar can also cause fatigue and muscle pain. A low fasting blood sugar may suggest hypoglycemia, although this is better diagnosed by taking a careful medical history. Likewise, normal fasting blood sugar does not rule out the presence of hypoglycemia.

At the time of your initial appointment, be sure to tell your doctor about any medications and supplements you are taking, and be honest about the amounts. It is very important *not* to forget to list your over-the-counter preparations. Analgesics such as acetaminophen and NSAIDs such as ibuprofen can raise liver enzymes. You should have both liver and kidney tests run if you take these medications. Elevated liver enzymes screen for the presence of hepatitis, another possible culprit for fatigue.

If your doctor suspects that you may have something other than fibromyalgia, or if you've never had a basic arthritis panel done, these tests should be done to rule out such things as rheumatoid arthritis and lupus. If you are a woman above the age of fifty, you can expect that your doctor will want to do a "sed rate." This test will detect a condition called *polymyalgia rheumatica*. Polymyalgia is *not* related to fibromyalgia, and is treated differently. Failure to diagnose and treat polymyalgia properly can result in blindness, so it is important to rule the possibility out.

From the above paragraphs you will have been reminded that there are no diagnostic blood tests for fibromyalgia. Blood tests are ordered only to ensure that nothing else is causing your symptoms. Only when other conditions have been ruled out can your doctor safely turn to the possibility that you have fibromyalgia.

The diagnosis of fibromyalgia is properly made in two parts. The doctor will begin by taking a detailed medical history and reviewing all of your body's systems. Since fibromyalgia causes such diverse symptoms as fatigue, depression, irritable bowel syndrome, irritable bladder, numbness, leg cramps, headaches, and palpitations, your doctor will want to ask you about these and other symptoms as well. Many doctors use check sheets to enumerate and keep track of the various symptoms. The two of you should try to establish a chronology of when your symptoms began, and construct a general time line of the progression of your illness. If you are diagnosed with fibromyalgia, this will prove helpful for both of you when you begin guaifenesin and start the reverse cycling.

After your doctor is satisfied that your symptoms and history suggest fibromyalgia, an examination will follow. He may not feel comfortable "mapping" as we do, but at the very least he will do a hands-on examination looking for the so-called "tender points." This search is especially revealing for those who think they only suffer from chronic fatigue syndrome, since it shows both patient and doctor the presence of the distinctive muscular findings of fibromyalgia. Finally, armed with the results of your blood tests, your history, systems review, and "tender point" or mapping examination, both you and your doctor should feel secure with your diagnosis.

❦ ADDRESS THE CARBOHYDRATE INTOLERANCE/ HYPOGLYCEMIA FACTOR

When you have been officially diagnosed with fibromyalgia, you have another important item to discuss with your doctor. If you are a woman, there is a forty percent chance that you have hypoglycemia or carbohydrate intolerance as well. It is imperative that you address this possibility before you go any further.

As we have explained in detail in the hypoglycemia chapter, there is no accurate blood test for hypoglycemia. The best way to decide whether or not you have hypoglycemia is to have your doctor take your history.

You will then be asked about two kinds of symptoms: acute and chronic. Normally the questioning begins with the acute symptoms because they are the easiest to identify. Acute symptoms are those that generally occur within three or four hours after eating, and are also common in the middle of the night. They are the symptoms that come on suddenly. Panic attacks, hand or inner shaking, sudden sweating, hunger headaches, heart pounding or rhythm irregularities, and severe anxieties are all acute symptoms but not all occur in every patient with hypoglycemia.

The chronic symptoms are more generalized ones. These are symptoms you may have all the time no matter what your blood sugar level is. They stem not from the drastic fall of blood sugar and the counterregulatory hormones, but from the metabolic fatigue caused by hypoglycemia. Headaches that are felt low and around the head like a rubber band are often related to blood sugar. If eating makes your symptoms go away, and you notice them more when you are hungry, blood sugar is the most likely culprit. Fatigue, irritability, nervousness, flushing, impaired memory and concentration, tight muscles, abdominal pain, bloating, gas, and diarrhea are among the chronic symptoms.

The doctor may also ask you general questions about your diet and your relationship with food. You may be asked about sugar or carbohydrate cravings, and about how you feel after you have eaten a meal heavy in sweets and starches. Again, even if you do not have *all* of the symptoms above, you may be carbohydrate-intolerant, and need to restrict your diet.

If you are hypoglycemic or carbohydrate-intolerant, you should begin our diet. Reread the hypoglycemia chapter of this book, and make a couple of copies of the diet. You will want one for your purse or wallet and one for your refrigerator door. You may want to keep one in your desk at work or in your car. Before you eat anything, make sure it is listed on the diet. *You must follow the diet perfectly for two months before you begin to experiment with unlisted foods.* Our diet is the only diet that we know that will control hypoglycemia. Other low-carbohydrate diets are constructed primarily for weight loss or for increasing energy and are not designed specifically to control hypoglycemia or carbohydrate intolerance.

Remember—if you need to lose weight, you belong on the *strict diet.* You are allowed to eat only the foods listed as part of this diet, which will control your hypoglycemia and carbohydrate cravings and allow you to lose weight. When you have lost the desired amount of weight and are ready for maintenance, it's time to add the foods from the liberal section.

If you are at a normal weight, you belong on the *liberal diet.* This diet will control your blood sugar if you pay attention to the limits next to each food item. It is important not to exceed them. The strict diet will *not* control your blood sugar any faster or better than the liberal one will. The only advantage of the strict diet is the weight reduction it produces; otherwise they are equally effective. If you are not carbohydrate-intolerant and are content with your weight, you might feel better if you avoided sugar and starch anyhow. This might give you a jump-start in energy for the reasons explained in the hypoglycemia chapter of this book.

If you are underweight, it is important that you eat the foods on the liberal diet. You will need to make sure that you eat enough of the allowed carbohydrates so that you do not lose weight. It is very difficult to gain weight and control your blood sugar simultaneously, so you will need to be extra careful. Make sure to eat your sugar-free bread and fruit as scheduled. Milk will also help to maintain your weight.

You will have to prepare for the diet by going to the market. Shopping will be slow until you get the hang of the diet, because you will have to read all the labels, so be sure to allow extra time to look at leisure. I suggest carrying a magnifying glass in your purse along with your copy of the diet. Pay special attention to the "Foods to Avoid Strictly" section when you are reviewing ingredients.

When you start the diet, you may feel more tired and irritable for the first several days. After about one week, your energy and symptoms will start to improve. At six weeks, you will have accrued most of the benefits from the diet—assuming that you have not cheated. If you have, it will take longer.

❧ MAP YOUR LUMPS AND BUMPS

If you want to be "mapped," and your physician does not feel confident enough to try it, you have several alternatives. Your doctor may be able to help you find a physical therapist, massage therapist, or chiropractor he or she knows and trusts. This is a convenient approach because you can have your maps sent to your doctor directly and he will be able to get feedback about your progress if he wants it. Make sure that you are referred to someone familiar with fibromyalgia.

In the unlikely event your doctor has no suggestions, ask your friends for a professional who does body work. When you make your appointment, don't forget to ask whether the person is knowledgeable about fibromyalgia. Local support groups may also be able to help you. It is actually much easier to find someone to agree to do the mapping than to prescribe the guaifenesin.

When you go to your first appointment, you should bring a copy of the "before treatment" illustration from page 154. This will visually describe to the mapper what we are trying to accomplish. The first "map" is very important, and it should be done before you begin your guaifenesin. If you are already taking the medicine, mapping will still have some benefit, since you should have it done at various times throughout your subsequent treatment. Each subsequent examination serves for comparison with the previous ones to ensure progress. We suggest that you do not skip this step.

Whether you visit a physical therapist, chiropractor, or massage therapist, all are accustomed to palpating muscles and tendons. They know what normal muscles feel like, and should be able to identify abnormal areas and draw these on the map. I draw the lesions as I feel them, using a darker color to illustrate harder spots. It is not mandatory for your examiner to use my system. He can devise his own method to ensure your lumps and bumps are recorded and graded for size and hardness. The only thing your mapper needs to know is that she or he should be mapping things that feel abnormal to him or her, and not the areas that hurt you when they are palpated. If she or he is especially interested in the process or has more than one patient on guaifenesin, there is a videotape available from Fibromeet in the Resources section of this book that shows Dr. St. Amand mapping a patient and explaining the process.

A tip for mapping is that the earliest site to reverse in most patients is the left vastus lateralis and rectus femoris (part of the thigh muscles, the quadriceps). Our sketches prominently display these two long, dark areas of spasm. When the left thigh is examined, the vastus lateralis is often described as one of the most tender areas of the body. Despite the apparent size of the lesions in these two muscles, when the proper dosage of guaifenesin is prescribed, they are among the first areas to release. We almost always find that they have partially or totally reversed with the *first month* of treatment. If you can only interest your doctor in a minimal form of monitoring, we strongly suggest that you have him or her examine these areas of the left thigh before and after treatment. If the drug dosage is correct at this site, it should prove adequate for all other areas as well. This simple examination will suggest that recovery is underway.

Be sure to make additional copies of your first map. You will want to make sure your doctor has one and that you have one in your own files. This paper is the road map for you, your doctors, and your physical therapists. It will illustrate the course you are taking. One day the lumps and bumps so graphically illustrated on this map will be just a memory. (Figure 6.1 shows a blank map.)

❧ ELIMINATE ALL SOURCES OF SALICYLATES

The last step before you begin your guaifenesin is extremely important. You must do a thorough search for salicylates in your medications, supplements, beauty products, and other topical applications. You must be very careful and check absolutely everything. Failure to do this correctly is the number-one reason for treatment failure. If you take shortcuts on this step, you will not give guaifenesin a fair chance to help you.

You may want to get a big garbage bag and gather up everything in the house that you use on your body. Set aside some time when you won't be disturbed, sit down with a dictionary and the lists in this book, and carefully do your work. You will end up with two piles: the products you can continue to use, and those you must get rid of. You should set aside any

Patient: _____ Date: _____

—FATIGUE   —OCCIPITAL HEADACHES   —DYSURIA

—IRRITABILITY   —DIZZINESS   —PUNGENT URINE

—NERVOUSNESS   —FAINTNESS   —BLADDER INFECTIONS

—DEPRESSION   —BLURRING VISION   —WEIGHT CHANGES

—INSOMNIA   —IRRITATED EYES   —BRITTLE NAILS

—IMPAIRED MEMORY   —NASAL CONGESTION   —ITCHING

—IMPAIRED CONCENTRATION   —ABNORMAL TASTES   —RASHES

—ANXIETY   —RINGING EARS   —HIVES

—SUGAR CRAVINGS   —NUMBNESS   —NEURODERMATITIS

—SALT CRAVINGS   —RESTLESS LEGS   —GROWING PAINS

—SWEATING   —LEG CRAMPS   —VULVODYNIA

—HUNGER TREMORS   —GAS   —PAINS

—PALPITATIONS   —BLOATING

—PANIC ATTACK   —CONSTIPATION

—FRONTAL HEADACHES   —DIARRHEA   **Figure 6.1**

questionable products, including those that don't list all their ingredients. Decide which manufacturers you need to call. Be sure to have a magnifying glass handy—the type on some packages is impossibly small! Remember: when products list only the *active ingredients,* you have to call the manufacturers for the inactive ones. Use no product in which you cannot identify every ingredient. If a product does not state whether the flavor it contains is synthetic or natural, call the company that manufactures it.

- Go through all your medications. This includes prescription and nonprescription medications such as pain-relievers, wart removers, suppositories, dandruff shampoos, and skin treatments. Make sure none of them contain plant parts, plant extracts, or salicylates by name. Check your over-the-counter topical medications such as cortisone creams. Every ingredient in vitamins and supplements should be carefully scrutinized. You will want to know the source of everything. All herbal supplements, such as St. John's wort and ginseng, must be discontinued right away. Do not assume because a product is a hormone such as melatonin or DHEA that an herb has not been added. If you are taking any medications, prescription or otherwise, that have a mint flavor be sure to check if natural mint is used. Pharmacists and on-line pharmacology information Web sites can assist you.

- Check every product in your bathroom. Mouthwashes, toothpastes, soaps, shampoos, conditioners, razors, shaving creams, deodorants, nasal sprays, lotions, toners, masks, ointments, suppositories, acne medications, and so on need to be looked at. Check all dental hygiene and gum care products for natural mint flavoring. Check lip balms and sunscreens. Many will contain salicylate by name, and some will contain aloe or other plants. Don't forget to check skin creams for the compound beta hydroxy. It is salicylic acid and will block your guaifenesin. Check everything in your first aid kit, especially topical muscle pain products and pain medications.

- Buy gardening gloves. Contact with plant oils and saps while gardening can deliver sufficient salicylate to block guaifenesin. If you dislike working in heavy gloves, try the thin latex variety used by doctors that can be found in most pharmacies. Be sure to keep your gloves handy so you can find them easily and wear them every time you work.

❧ BEGIN TAKING GUAIFENESIN

Get a prescription for plain guaifenesin from your doctor. (All guaifenesin is "LA," or long acting.) When you pick up your prescription, make sure there is only one ingredient listed— guaifenesin. There should be only one number following the name. It will either be 600 or 1200. If you see two numbers, for example a 600/120, you may have been given the wrong medication. (Two numbers generally indicate that there are two ingredients present.) Double-check with the pharmacist if you are not sure from the label whether or not you have the plain compound. There are many brands and shades of guaifenesin tablets, such as blue, green, teal, and white, because there are many generics—no patent remains on the drug. Don't worry if you get a different one from time to time. But you should always check with the pharmacist or your doctor if you are not sure what you have been given.

Guaifenesin has about a twelve-hour action, so you should take it twice a day. Some people who require higher doses take their guaifenesin three times a day—especially if it bothers their stomach a little. But for most people, twice a day in divided doses is fine. (The doses don't have to be evenly divided. For example, if your dose is three pills a day, you can take two in the morning and one at night, or one three times a day.)

❦ FIND YOUR DOSE

It is important to be systematic and hold at each dose for the specified amount of time. It will be much easier for you and your doctor if you follow this part of the protocol exactly. We cannot emphasize this enough. If you are not methodical about establishing your dose it will be much more difficult later on. Tempting as it may be to raise or lower your dose on a daily basis, *don't do it!* The person you will confuse the most will be yourself.

You may get advice from other patients or support group members to raise or lower your dose based on how you feel at any given moment. Ignore them. *Do not change your dosage of guaifenesin or any other medication without talking to your doctor.* If you have doubts about your dosage, pay careful attention to your symptoms and get a map made to be sure you are reversing properly. Sometimes only a map can tell you where you stand. When it comes to your health, why create a guessing game? Follow our instructions and those of your physician.

When you begin taking guaifenesin, it's a good idea to keep track of what happens. We suggest a small desk calendar, one with space enough to write a few words every day. Keep your notations simple; this will make it easier to decipher the patterns of good and bad days. Possible entries might read: "headache 1/2 day" or "more energy in the A.M." or "back better." Simple notes such as "shoulder stopped hurting" or "neck very sore" are of great help. It's tempting to rate days on a scale of one to ten for all symptoms, especially pain. This may seem like a good system in the beginning, but eventually you will realize that these numbers have become progressively more difficult to compare. Once you are experiencing runs of several good weeks, it is difficult to remember the severity of earlier cycles. Down the line, your worst day may be considerably better than your good days were before you started your treatment.

With your doctor's consent, start by taking 300 mg of guaifenesin twice a day. This usually requires breaking 600 mg tablets in half. (Some drugstore labels may caution against this, but there is no problem with doing so.) In our opinion, there is no advantage to starting out with a dosage lower than 300 mg twice a day. We have seen only a very few patients reverse with lower amounts. If you are concerned that you are "sensitive to medications," 300 mg twice a day is a very low dose for guaifenesin.

Take 300 mg twice a day for one week. If you become distinctly worse, that is probably your dosage. Always remember that when you reach your dose, your symptoms will get worse. If you are tired, you will be more tired. If you ache, you will ache more. Symptoms that were mild or barely noticeable before may bother you now. Because symptoms are more acute in reversal, you may develop some pains or aches that seem new to you. This is because you must exceed your threshold before you feel pain, and past cycles may have been gentle ones, below your perception level in that area.

If you do not feel distinctly worse during this first week, speak to your doctor about doubling your dose to one 600 mg tablet twice a day, or a total of 1200 mg a day. You will usually notice an exacerbation of your symptoms within ten to fourteen days if this proves adequate. If you again notice no appreciable difference in the intensity of your fibromyalgia after another three weeks, again ask permission to raise your dose to 1800 mg a day. This amount of medication has proved sufficient to initiate reversal in ninety percent of our patients. As in the preceding steps, almost all patients will feel worse when they attain their required dosage.

If you hold at 1800 mg a day for one month and nothing changes, neither worse nor better days, you should again speak with your doctor and ask to raise your dosage to 1200 mg twice a day. This amount proves adequate for over ninety-five percent of our patients. Just as before, hold this dose for another month. If there is no change in your condition, you may be one of the rare people who require an even higher dosage, 3600 or even 4800 mg per day. (See figure 6.2.) However, because success is so high at 2400 mg, it is time for another very thorough search for a blocking salicylate. At this point it is common for us to ask our patients to "bag your groceries" and bring in all their topicals and supplements for our inspection. If nothing turns up and their map hasn't changed, then we typically raise their dose again.

Finding the proper dosage may not be easy for some people. A small number of patients, possibly five percent, will have only minimal symptoms during their reverse cycles. Without a mapping to confirm that improvement has begun, such individuals might raise their guaifenesin dosage well beyond what they actually need. This is why it is a good idea to map before increasing the medication. For those few patients who improve without getting noticeably worse, an improving map is the signal to go slowly and patiently await the appearance of good days.

🐚 REMAPPING ON GUAIFENESIN

It is best to revisit the same person who did your initial mapping so that the techniques will be comparable. At all times during your treatment, remapping is very important, since changes become progressively more subtle. When only a few areas remain to be cleared, only tiny improvements may be felt, as more difficult tissues such as the tendons are now being purged. Because these structures have poorer blood supplies, guaifenesin penetration is much slower.

We map our patients at every visit. After we are certain about their dosage, we can gradually stretch their appointments out—first to three, then six, and finally to twelve months. Lumps and bumps should get progressively smaller, softer, or more mobile. Some of the larger areas, such as those at the hips or tops of the shoulders, will often split into one or two smaller areas. At the same time, patients tell us about their subjective symptoms and observations. We hide our old maps and refer to them only after we have completed the new one. This is as objective a procedure as is possible in the treatment of fibromyalgia. You and your physician should agree on the frequency of mapping—whatever schedule allows you both the maximum level of comfort. Don't overlook the fact that an important benefit of mapping is that it can quickly detect a sa-

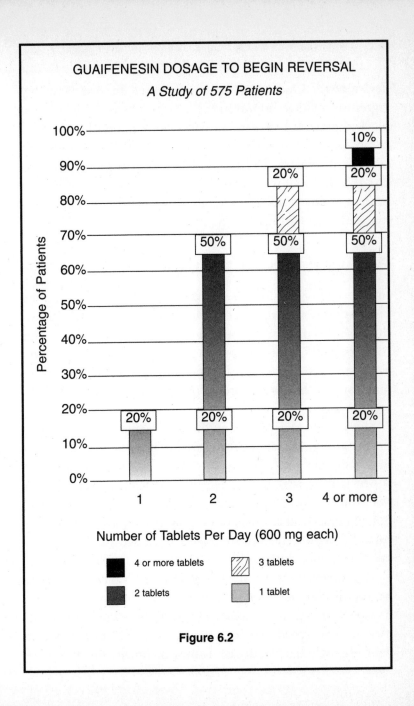

GUAIFENESIN DOSAGE TO BEGIN REVERSAL

A Study of 575 Patients

Figure 6.2

licylate block. Once a map has shown initial improvement, any regression of that improvement will be obvious. Since most blocked patients begin to feel worse fairly rapidly, their added complaints and their deteriorating map alert them to recheck all their products. We have used this system for many years and it is the way we actually discovered some of the hidden sources of salicylates. (Figure 6.3 shows maps of a patient before and after starting treatment.)

❦ HAVE AN ANNUAL EVALUATION

In our state of California, a physician, by law, must examine patients every year in order to write a prescription. These annual or semiannual visits permit us to reevaluate and map our patients. This confirms progress and insures that previous clearing is sustained. At this time your doctor will be able to monitor your health and order any blood tests he or she thinks appropriate.

Eventually each patient asks how long one should continue to take guaifenesin after getting well. The answer to this question is simple: guaifenesin works only when you are taking it. When you stop taking it, the genetic defect that caused your symptoms is unchanged, and your disease will return. It will not come back all at once, or even overnight, but it will come back. Rather dependably, the dose that caused your first reversal cycle is your dose for life.

For many there is a strong temptation to try a lower dose or stop guaifenesin altogether when their symptoms are gone. If you increased your medication during the course of treatment just to speed up the reversal, lowering your intake to your original effective dosage is proper. But if you drop your

These maps show results in a 39-year-old woman who has been on guaifenesin 600 mg bid. She was initially seen and mapped on November 7, 1995, but did not begin treatment until May 14, 1996. The results you see, therefore, are the effect of medication over a span of 10 months (from May 14, 1996 to March 11, 1997).

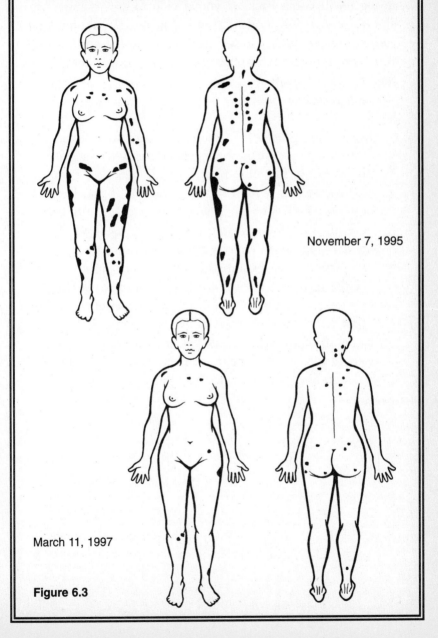

November 7, 1995

March 11, 1997

Figure 6.3

dosage too low, below your therapeutic level, your fibromyalgia will come back. If you decide to try to lower the amount anyway, use a calendar and make notations about your various symptoms. If you see that you are losing ground, and your symptoms are returning, resume your proper dosage and hold the line thereafter.

One patient advises:

> Just do the protocol. Let time pass and stick it out. Don't worry so much about whether it is working or not working. Let time pass. Nobody gets well from guaifenesin in a week or even a month. If you have been sick for a long time, which it seems most of us have, then it takes *time* to get well. *Time.* Quit watching the clock and live each day to the degree that you can. Try to think of something other than illness. . . . Let the guai work. I was constantly tempted to raise [my dosage]. Did I? No. For me it was better to not think so much. I just tried to live. I concentrated and had faith that if others could get well on this protocol, I could too. . . . It is a path of stealth health. You just wake up one morning, and there you are.
>
> —*Gloria, Florida*

Part II

❧

UNDERSTANDING THE MANY FACETS OF FIBROMYALGIA

Part I of this book, which you've just read, provides a general overview of the disease of fibromyalgia, a little history, and a little bit of our experiences. It also explains about the medication we use and why we think it works, and outlines the treatment protocol. So what's left for Parts II and III?

Part II, which you're about to start, goes into a lot more detail about fibromyalgia, and each of the chapters deals with a cluster of symptoms, or a "syndrome." Each of these will help you understand your body and how fibromyalgia affects it. The chapters also provide some solutions for coping and controlling your symptoms until the guaifenesin makes them go away. We've also included quotations from guaifenesin patients about their experiences and yours. We hope you'll find those interesting and you will understand that you are far from alone.

There's no question that knowledge is power, especially

in medicine. The more you know and the more your doctor knows, the better off you are. When you go to the store and buy something, you're paying for a material object. Doctors, on the other hand, have only experience and wisdom to share, and that's what this next section is—knowledge we want to share with you.

So now that you've had time to digest the basics, let's move ahead and learn more about what the disease is doing to your body, and how you can fight back using guaifenesin.

Chapter 7

❧

Genitourinary Syndromes

Over the years we have learned that the bladder, urethra, and vaginal tract have all shared in some of the most overwhelming symptoms of fibromyalgia. It took us several years to make the connection between these intense cycles and the basic disease. At times, symptoms in these areas are so oppressive that patients are hardly aware of their intestinal or musculoskeletal problems. For this reason the search for relief usually begins with urologists or gynecologists who become increasingly frustrated by their inability to help their patients. Because fibromyalgia is not part of their expertise, the larger disease of their patients remains undiagnosed. Desperately seeking some form of relief, these patients are too often referred for surgeries that do not help them.

❧ BLADDER

Early in our work, it became apparent that many fibromyalgic women suffer from recurrent, problematic vaginal and bladder symptoms. Approximately twenty-five percent of female fibromyalgics have had three or more bladder infections in their lifetimes. A few women tell us they have had fifty or more attacks of this cystitis and many more episodes of painful urination when there was no infection. Routine urinalysis in healthy patients often shows all varieties and shapes of amorphous crystals, most of which are composed of calcium phosphate (some are calcium oxalate or other compounds). You will recall that in fibromyalgics, the entire body participates in trying to get rid of the accumulated phosphates. Acid secretions in tears, saliva, sweat, bowel, and vagina all help, but most of it is excreted in the urine. Excess phosphate combines in the bladder with calcium or magnesium to form crystals in the urine, while in other body fluids it remains in solution without forming precipitates. Crystals in the urine settle to the lowest portion of the bladder, near the opening of the urethra, where they concentrate and aggregate. During the next urination, this collection of crystals exits with the first part of the urinary flow and acts like an abrasive on the delicate lining, the mucosa. If this scraping is sufficiently severe, the integrity of the membranes is compromised, and if the membranes are broken, bacteria can penetrate. The short female urethra—the tube leading out of the bladder—presents only a small distance for infection to travel, resulting in cystitis. This is why fibromyalgic women suffer far more problems with their urinary tract than men or normal individuals. (See figure 7.1.)

Cystitis—Infection of the bladder. Symptoms include a constant urge to urinate, pain above the pubic bone, burning, searing urine, and, upon urination, producing only a small amount of urine. Antibiotics are commonly prescribed to treat the infection, as well as local analgesics that work on the urinary tract.

The same problem often arises from intercourse. Most women know about "honeymoon cystitis," and for many it is true that the bulk of their infections occurred at times when they were more sexually active. The accumulated crystals in the bladder permit damage to the wall caused by the friction of strokes from the penis.

Some patients have taken antibiotics steadily for a year or more in an attempt to eradicate the problem. Others describe attacks where they experienced all of the symptoms of cystitis but no infection could be documented even with a urine culture. They had the same burning sensations during urination, sometimes for only a few hours and at other times for days. Frequent and powerful urges to urinate often produced only dribbling and scanty amounts of urine. Occasionally, blood or pus was present either to the naked eye or, more often, only microscopically. Without a urine culture, even the most chronically affected patient can be fooled by the symptoms, believing there is an infection where none, in fact, exists. Since many of these same women develop yeast infections or diarrhea from the antibiotics used to treat infection, it is well worth the small expense of a urinalysis to make sure that an antibiotic is necessary.

Mechanism of Bladder Infection or Irritation

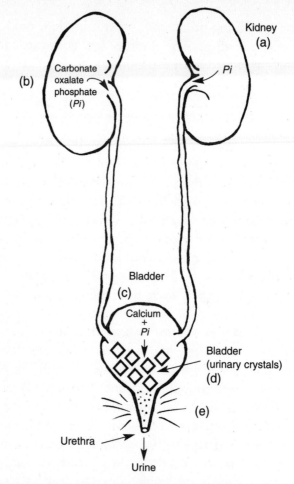

(a) Kidneys retain too much but eliminate some phosphate.
(b) Kidneys release oxalates and carbonates (*anions* that, like phosphates, have two negative charges).
(c) In the bladder the anions combine mostly with calcium (*cations* that, like magnesium, have two positive charges).
(d) The combining of cations and anions forms crystals that settle to the bottom of the bladder.
(e) At the next urination the crystals scrape the bladder neck and the urethra, exposing the lining to infection.

Figure 7.1

> *Cystoscopy*—A procedure done in a doctor's office, in which the urinary tract is viewed through a cystoscope inserted through the urethra and up into the bladder. Through this fiber-optic scope, the doctor can examine the lining and structure of these organs. A patient is usually given a local anesthetic or a mild tranquilizer to help with the discomfort.

Many women have undergone thorough investigations by competent urologists. Repeated urine cultures only occasionally found bacterial causes. Most of these patients eventually underwent one or more cystoscopies in a futile search for anatomical defects. When none was found, biopsies of the bladder lining and deeper wall structures were taken and examined microscopically. The normal results of these procedures usually caused frustration for the patient and the urologist. At most, all that could be found was a small accumulation of white blood cells—not sufficient findings for a significant conclusion.

> I had always had vulvar pain, suffered from bladder infections for two weeks, then yeast infections for two weeks and back to bladder, and so on. I had constant infections for over eleven years. I was given a cystoscope and a cystogram, because the doctors thought I had cancer. Nothing showed up. I had a urologist and an ob/gyn mystified.
>
> —*Cyndi S., Dallas*

Interstitial cystitis—A disease defined by the absence of positive tests for other bladder conditions, manifested by bladder and pelvic pain and the constant urge to urinate which produces only a small amount of urine.

These normal or inconsequential findings usually earn the now commonly heard diagnosis of "interstitial cystitis." Symptoms of this condition include pelvic or pubic area pain and an urgent sensation to urinate that is so strong that some patients say they have tried to void fifty to eighty times a day. Urine cultures are routinely negative. Vaginal and rectal pain are also common. Sometimes hard spasms occur in the area between the vagina and rectum, the perineum. Interstitial cystitis is diagnosed more rarely in male patients, where it is often misdiagnosed as nonbacterial prostatitis, or prostatodynia.

Sufferers have shortened the name to "IC" and formed excellent support groups all over the world. It is estimated that some 450,000 people, ninety percent of whom are women, have been diagnosed with interstitial cystitis in the United States. The average age of diagnosis is forty, about the same as the average person diagnosed with fibromyalgia. Both of the two large IC organizations, the ICN (the Interstitial Cystitis Network) and the ICA (the Interstitial Cystitis Association) have noticed that their groups have a very large number of fibromyalgics, and now include information on fibromyalgia in their brochures and on their Web sites. Fibromyalgia, irritable bowel syndrome, and vulvodynia are the most common concurrent conditions with IC, according to patient surveys published by these groups. Both the ICA and the ICN give out dietary suggestions and other hints for controlling symptoms, and are listed in the Resources section of this book.

The diet is, generally speaking, one that restricts caffeine, alcohol, and foods high in acid or spices. Patients who use guaifenesin can continue to use medications that numb the bladder such as Pyridium or its over-the-counter version, phenazopyridine hydrochloride. Some relief can also be obtained from drinking half a teaspoon of baking soda in a six-ounce glass of water three times a day to neutralize the acidity of the urine. Cranberry juice or tablets are sometimes offered to patients to prevent urinary tract infections. Cranberry juice or vitamin C may raise urinary acidity—although this is no longer thought to be the mechanism by which they work. But if urination is already painful, this increased acidity makes symptoms worse. Guaifenesin users should not use cranberry tablets because they may block the guaifenesin. Patients who are being treated for bladder problems should carefully check any medications they are taking before beginning guaifenesin. *Both Urised and Prosed contain phenyl salicylate, and will therefore block guaifenesin.* Antidepressants are also prescribed for this condition, as is a newer drug, Elmiron (pentosan polysulfate), which provides a coating on the bladder lining, thus easing the symptoms of IC. It will not block guaifenesin.

When you're having an attack, the constant pain . . . the fear of sex making more pain is debilitating. It weighs down your life, your lightness, destroys spontaneity, makes you standoffish with the man you love because you just don't want to have to explain you're having problems *again*. That part is bad, but the symptoms that you live with night and day are even worse: never sleeping through a night, having to sleep on the outside of every bed, always worrying whether there will be a bathroom close by, stopping often on car trips, dodging into fast-food places, hoping they won't catch you not buying anything and telling you the rest room is only for customers.

—*C.C., La Jolla, CA*

Guaifenesin eventually clears IC complaints. Bladder symptoms initially intensify and cycle in the same way as the other symptoms of fibromyalgia. Reversal attacks are progressively less and less severe with each cycle, until they disappear completely. When painful urination (dysuria) begins during treatment, patients should immediately start drinking extra fluid to lessen the severity of the attack. They can also add bicarbonate tablets (available over the counter in pharmacies) three or four times a day to lessen urinary acidity.

🐚 VULVAR PAIN

As senior gynecologist with special training and expertise in vulvar disease, I have been striving to help women with the enigmatic disorder called vulvodynia, and its most common subset, vulvar vestibulitis. In recent years there has been increasing appreciation of other conditions reported as commonly associated with vulvodynia, such as irritable bowel syndrome, fibromyalgia, and interstitial cystitis. In my own practice at Scripps Clinic and Research Foundation I've discovered that fibromyalgia is at least three times as common in vulvodynia patients as in the general population. I've also noted that vulvodynia tends not to respond to therapy until the underlying fibromyalgia is treated. . . . Dr. St. Amand has done ground-breaking work in the evaluation and treatment of fibromyalgia as opposed to medications that only reduce or help control symptoms. His research, and that of those who follow in his footsteps, will permit fibromyalgia to become merely a painful memory for patients and their spouses. I salute his effort.

> —*John Willems, M.D., FRCSC, FACOG,*
> *Head, Division of Ob/Gyn, Scripps Clinic and*
> *Research Foundation, La Jolla, CA*

Vulvodynia or vulvar pain syndrome—Severe pain, burning, and/or itching in the vulvar (the vulva is the area of the female's external genitalia) area. This area is extremely sensitive to touch, and may or may not be red and visibly irritated. Vulvar Vestibulitis Syndrome (VVS) is less common, and applies to women who have pain only in the vestibule, a smaller area than the vulva.

Many fibromyalgia women complain of severe sensitivity caused by irritation of the inner vaginal lips near the opening. This sometimes occurs only after intercourse, but often with-

Internal Female Reproductive Organs

Showing the interweave of muscles and organs responsible for pelvic pain.

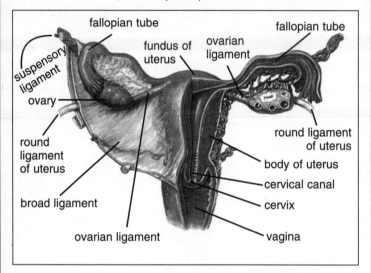

The Vulva

Showing the areas affected by vulvar pain (vulvodynia) and vulvar vestibulitis.

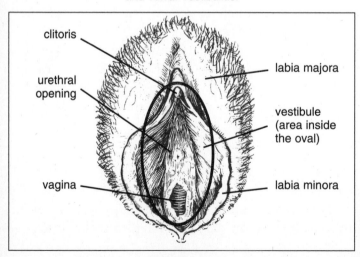

Figure 7.2

out apparent provocation, resulting in chronic, eventually over-whelming symptoms. Wearing tight jeans, nylon underwear, or pantyhose can make symptoms flare, and the constant pain is intolerable. Prolonged rides in cars or aircraft trigger increased pain simply from clothing seams pressing into and chafing the vaginal area. More often than not, these patients also suffer si-multaneously from the recurrent cystitis we described above. For others, though, this burning is not due to bladder prob-lems, but instead comes from urine pouring over irritated, vul-val tissue. Steady pressure and aching in the suprapubic area is also suggestive of a bladder infection. Fibromyalgia also regu-larly affects the inguinal ligaments, the cordlike structures that connect the hip to the pubic bone. These constricted ligaments steadily tug at nerves, leading to a steady aching sensed as deep pelvic pain. Occasionally, spasms (charley horse) in the per-ineal area or the vaginal muscles and ligaments will produce in-tense pain.

Women with vulvar pain syndrome often have irritable bowel syndrome as well. In fact, so often do they occur together that we have realized that they are part and parcel of the same disease. We have therefore added these presumably separate en-tities to the growing list of so-called syndromes and isolated symptoms that we fit into the larger, single disease, fibromyalgia.

A few years ago we began working closely with a nation-wide group, the Vulvar Pain Foundation, headquartered in Graham, North Carolina. This group is dedicated to helping women with vulvodynia. Somewhat like fibromyalgia, vulvo-dynia is too often a diagnosis of exclusion. Exhaustive testing is usually done, and if other conditions such as infections or nerve or dermatological damage are not found, the diagnosis of vulvodynia is made. The diagnosis is usually delayed until a woman is in her forties, although it can occur at any age. Studies show that between 150,000 and 200,000 women in the United States suffer from this disease. It was quickly obvious to us that this is an underestimation, in view of the number of fibromyalgic women we see who suffer with the same symptoms.

Doctor Clive Solomons, Ph.D., a biochemist working in Denver, is conducting ongoing research on methods to ease or control the symptoms of vulvodynia. He has focused especially on the effects of urinary oxalates as direct irritants to the labia. Oxalates are readily absorbed from foods and are also produced during normal metabolism. Doctor Solomons has studied urine specimens obtained at various times of the day and found high levels of oxalates in women with vulvodynia.[21] Our observations support his findings indirectly, because we documented an increase of thirty percent in oxalate excretion after the initiation of guaifenesin treatment in some fibromyalgics.

Doctor Solomons's treatment begins with putting patients on a low-oxalate diet which relieves symptoms by lowering levels in the urine. The Vulvar Pain Foundation has published a cookbook to facilitate adherence to the diet. Under Doctor Solomons's guidance, the foundation also suggests that women with vulvodynia add calcium citrate. This binds oxalates within the digestive tract and prevents absorption. We have listed the address of the foundation and its Web site in the Resources section of this book.

Oxalate—A chemical found in the human body as part of the energy production cycle. It is excreted in the urine, and is known as a topical irritant which can cause burning in the tissues. Foods of plant origin, such as fruits and vegetables, are high in oxalates.

Women with the debilitating condition of vulvodynia are fortunate to have another strong support group, the National Vulvodynia Association in Silver Spring, Maryland, founded in 1994. It has an excellent Web site and, like the Vulvar Pain Foundation, is also working diligently to help women and their partners to cope with the symptoms of this condition. Women with vulvodynia have been deeply conditioned to expect excruciating and long-lasting pain during and following intercourse. They can become afraid of simple cuddling for fear that even this bit of solace might lead to more. Desire is so dulled that lubrication is minimal and the mere thought of making love arouses recall of an intolerable sensation we describe as "sandpapering" the labia. Relationships are severely tested. High incidences of separation and divorce occur within this group. Some women freely admit that they have avoided forming a meaningful relationship knowing that they would eventually be expected to perform sexually. A typical story appears below:

Prior to the guaifenesin treatments and my proper diagnosis, the most debilitating pain I would experience was the vulvar pain. The muscle pain could be significantly minimized with pain relievers but not the vulvar pain. In 1989 the vulvar pain became extreme and frequent. It was so severe at times that I would miss work. Because of this pain, I avoided intercourse with my husband and rejected the thought of having a baby.

My only relief from pain was warm baths, but I could not live in the bathtub all the time, so I sought help from my family physician. Even though [he] . . . was aware of my other symptoms (acne, muscle pain, insomnia) he focused on each symptom as a separate medical condition and sent me to a variety of specialists. Since he did not focus on the body as a whole and was ignorant of the existence of fibromyalgia, he did not connect my cycles of muscle pain, and fatigue . . . with my vulvar pain.

During the first few weeks of taking the guaifenesin I did experience vulvar pain an average of about two out of ten days, and the pain was severe. As I continued to take the guaifenesin, both the frequency and the severity of the pain decreased. . . . Since January 1995 I have not missed work due to fibromyalgia or vulvar pain. I am not fearful of sexual intercourse, and maybe one day I will even think about having a baby.

—*Angela Domnikov, Torrance, CA, letter printed in the* Vulvar Pain Newsletter

Both the foundation and the association have observed a strong tie between fibromyalgia and vulvar pain. They do not yet acquiesce in our belief that nearly all women with vulvodynia have fibromyalgia, but they are certainly pursuing this link. I believe that this official recognition would be an obvious medical bonanza for these women, since the actual, underlying cause of their illness would be remediable.

Another pioneer in the field of vulvodynia is John Willems, M.D., Chief of Obstetrics and Gynecology at Scripps Clinic in La Jolla, California. He has contributed greatly to the education of both women and the medical profession about this condition. As we have already stated, patients with fibromyalgia turn to the medical specialist who seems most appropriate to treat the dominant symptoms of their illness. Doctor Willems has diagnosed many patients with both the vulvar pain syndrome and fibromyalgia. Before we met, he had already found that about twenty-five percent of his vulvodynia patients had fibromyalgia. This is a significant number since, as a gynecologist, fibromyalgia is not a diagnosis he would have normally considered in his field of expertise.

This blatant assault on these women's fundamental quality of life has driven many to embrace drastic "cures." Those who had sought relief with various creams and lotions were the least harmed by treatment. Fortunately, they suffered only a wounded purse. Others submitted to repeated injections into the painful areas of local anesthetics or alcohol given with synthetic cortisones. More shocking and horrifying are the reports on file at the Vulvar Pain Foundation that tell of the unsuccessful and sometimes mutilating surgeries women have undergone. Parts of the labia or vagina are often removed in an attempt to eliminate painful sites. Most of these surgeries were followed by a recurrence of symptoms and, worse still, left scarring that sometimes even increased them. Unfortunately, surgery remains "the thing to do" too soon and too often. Doctor Willems has had considerable success in decreasing the symptoms of vulvar pain with his treatment protocol that advocates using topical estradiol to thicken and rebuild the thinned, vulvar tissue.[22] He is outspoken in maintaining that

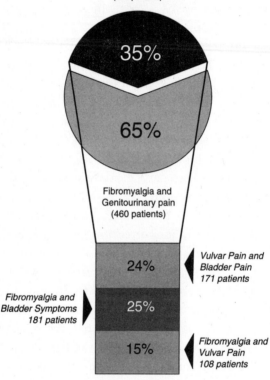

FIBROMYALGIA, VULVAR PAIN, AND BLADDER SYMPTOMS

Study of 712 Consecutive Female Patients

FIBROMYALGIA ONLY
(252 patients)

35%

65%

Fibromyalgia and
Genitourinary pain
(460 patients)

Vulvar Pain and
Bladder Pain
171 patients

24%

Fibromyalgia and
Bladder Symptoms
181 patients

25%

15%

Fibromyalgia and
Vulvar Pain
108 patients

Women with Fibromyalgia—65% have genitourinary pain

Figure 7.3

surgery should be the last resort and for only a small number of patients. Estradiol cream should be made with an oil base without plant derivatives when it is to be used by women taking guaifenesin. Compounding pharmacists can easily make such a preparation. Some compounding pharmacies are listed in the back of this book. Scripps clinic is listed in the Resources section.

We have known and treated several thousand patients with fibromyalgia. Few of them have known more pitiful symptoms than those who have had to endure the intense discomfort and mental anguish of vulvodynia.

> I have suffered from vulvar pain since 1990. I went everywhere for help. I even flew to Michigan for laser surgery from a now infamous doctor. I hooked up with the Vulvar Pain Foundation and found out about the low-oxalate diet and citrate. I began this treatment and got a little better. I added Estrace cream per Dr. Willems at Scripps Clinic in La Jolla, CA. . . . I found out about Dr. St. Amand from the VP Foundation and read up on him. I firmly believed that I did not have FMS because I didn't have the body aches and pains. But as I read through the symptoms of FMS I was astounded. I was reading my life's history. I began the guaifenesin, and the first thing that left me was the vulvar pain. Now I do indeed have the general aches and pains (but that's due to the cycling). I also realize that I have a high pain tolerance and just tolerated the aches. I cycled fairly quickly. Dr. St. Amand recently mapped me, and I'm almost cleared out!
>
> —*Mary B., Alabama*

❦

Chapter 8

The Irritable Bowel Syndrome:
Fibrogut

It is not unusual for some fibromyalgics to suffer predominantly from abdominal symptoms. Many physicians have difficulty accurately assessing the problem within the abdominal organs unless the patient's history leads them in the proper direction. For example, we see individuals who have dull but steady aching in some part of the abdomen and tenderness from our hand pressure during the examination. This provides very little evidence as to what is really going on inside and makes a proper diagnosis extremely difficult. By the time these patients appear in our office, they have usually undergone many tests. A typical history goes like this.

Because of persistent aching or even more intense pain, the primary physician does a basic work-up consisting of his examination, X rays, and the standard blood tests. If no abnormality is discovered, he refers the patient to a gastroenterologist. This specialist reviews the lab reports and confirms that everything so far seems to be functioning normally. His or her manual examination also reveals nothing unusual. Often, an ultrasound is then performed, which shows that the liver, spleen, and gall-bladder appear to be structurally normal. This may next lead to an endoscopy of the esophagus, stomach, and upper part of the small intestine. A colonoscopy may follow and simply add to the growing list of normal findings if all symptoms are caused by fibromyalgia. Our perfectly tested subject is now informed that no serious problem has been located. Finally, by process of elimination, the patient is given the diagnosis of "irritable bowel syndrome" (IBS). However, specialists specialize and therefore tend to remain in their field of expertise. They may fail to see the broader picture and do not realize they are actually facing a more widespread, total-body disease. Too infrequently will a correlation be drawn between the IBS and fibromyalgia.

Ultrasound—High-frequency sound waves are passed by a transducer through the area of the body to be studied, to make an image of solid organs such as the liver. These waves cannot pass through bones or make images of gas.

Endoscopy—This procedure is done with a fiber-optic instrument enabling direct visual examination. A long narrow tube is inserted through the mouth, down the back of the throat into the esophagus, down into the stomach and into the duodenum, the first part of the small intestine.

Colonoscopy—To examine the colon, a similar but longer endoscope (colonoscope) is inserted rectally and passed upward. The doctor then withdraws it slowly, as each part of the intestine and rectum is examined. This procedure is usually done in a doctor's office or hospital "GI lab" with the patient mildly sedated. If only the lower portion of the colon is to be examined, a shorter instrument is used for a "Sigmoidoscopy."

Over the years, many other names have been used to describe IBS, such as spastic colon, mucous colitis, and functional bowel disease. Recently, another name has crept into our medical jargon, "the leaky gut syndrome." I believe these are all names for the same condition. Most of the terms describe what physicians inaccurately believe causes the condition. For example, the term colitis means inflammation of the colon. There is no inflammation with IBS and it does not progress to a more serious disease or cancer. There are no visible anatomical or measurable biochemical abnormalities.

As in all other facets of fibromyalgia, women are affected by IBS in far greater numbers than are men, and the symptoms are worse premenstrually. The disease may begin at any age and often strikes children or young adults.

Since my teenage years I have had stomach pain and cramping. . . . My general practitioner would say it was "a little gastritis." He would prescribe an antacid and send me home with a pat on the back. I suffered like this for about ten or twelve years. . . . I went to a very eminent gastroenterologist. . . . He pronounced "irritable bowel syndrome." When I asked him what I could do for it he said "Nothing. Just stay away from green vegetables." . . . I also experienced insomnia and some muscle pain since I was a teen. I had no idea they were all related to FMS. A few years ago the FMS came on with a vengeance, and after seeking a diagnosis for about nine months I finally found a doctor who told me I have FMS with gastroesophageal reflux.

—*Marie N.*

Sixty percent of our fibromyalgics have IBS. There are many symptoms within the complex of IBS. Not all patients have every symptom. Sometimes there is intermittent difficulty in swallowing. Acid can reflux back up the esophagus from the stomach and cause heartburn, which is an acid taste or an actual chemical burn. The acid irritation may cause esophageal spasms and produce chest pain that can closely mimic cardiac pain. This is labeled gastroesophageal reflux or GER. Waves of nausea sometimes appear out of nowhere. They can last for hours or for only a few seconds but in frequent, repetitive waves. Gas and bloating are among the most common complaints, but just as high on the patient's list is frequent constipation alternating with diarrhea.

These symptoms may lead physicians to administer a battery of skin allergy tests, and the patients are then told they have multiple food sensitivities. There would follow an attempt to confirm these skin findings using a series of very expensive blood tests. Though the tests may be correct in their assessment, patients sometimes tell us they have no problem when they eat many of the supposedly offending foods. When

I hear this, I encourage patients to do an eating test using a small amount of one item at a time and let their gastrointestinal tract tell them if they really must avoid that food. Each food can be tried in sequence and, if sensitivity truly exists, symptoms get decidedly worse. Only then would one really have to stop eating that particular ingredient. This is the true proof of sensitivity.

Constipation and diarrhea can take turns in rapid shifts. However, it is not rare to have one problem for months or years and suddenly have the other one enter the picture. This combination, but particularly the diarrhea, can lead to stool testing for candida (yeast) or parasites. Stool examinations are not for the novice technician. It takes the practiced eye of a skilled expert to avoid being deceived into thinking that certain food residues are cysts or parasites. It is especially difficult to avoid errors since a certain amount of yeast is normal in stool specimens. Repeatedly, patients have undergone many varieties of herbal purgings, colonic cleansings, or heavy cathartic "washouts," all in the vain attempt to clean out something that was never there. Still others have spent months or years on antifungal (yeast) medications, such as Mycostatin or fluconazole, without experiencing a change in their symptoms.

How does it feel physically? I described it to a friend this way: "Imagine you are just recovering from a bad case of the stomach flu, where you're better but still shaky and not sure how loose your bowels still are. Now imagine you're going to try to carry on a normal life, and pretend you're fine. And imagine every day is like this." It's hard, it's uncomfortable, and the emotional component is hard too. Cramping, urgency, a feeling of "looseness," burning pain in the lower back, nausea, acid reflux, shakiness, weak knees. These are all symptoms I associate with IBS.

—*R.A., California*

The irritable bowel syndrome is really a cascade of sequential problems. These include irritation of the rectum, internal or external hemorrhoids, fissures, and occasional, bloody stools. When a patient is constipated, it is common for the lower bowel to form mucus. The colon responds with mucus, just as nasal and bronchial membranes do when they are irritated. In the case of the colon, the irritant is the bowel movement that has hardened during the long wait to exit. The stony hard stool presses against the wall of the lower colon, where it causes spasm which causes pain in the lower, left side of the abdomen, in the sigmoid colon. The colon lining, the mucous membrane, produces its mucus in an effort to coat and lubricate the abrasive effect of the stool and help the next bowel movement to slide out more easily. The movement is sometimes accompanied by a stained, mucous string that somewhat resembles a long worm. If the beginning part of the stool is hard enough, the lining of the rectum could also be scratched and caused to bleed. This is particularly true if a hard food particle is imbedded on the surface of the stool. The presence of these hard stools, day after day, causes patients to strain in an attempt to move their bowels. The rocky stool can push a rectal vein ahead of it, similar to a rising wave, and create the rectal protrusion we call a hemorrhoid. When hard bits tear the rectal lining to produce bleeding, the examining physician may find the source and, in medical parlance, diagnose a "rectal fissure."

The cause of the IBS symptoms is fibromyalgia. Cells of the gastrointestinal tract cannot form sufficient energy. The three muscle layers of the intestinal wall also contract and become dysfunctional, just as the skeletal muscles do. The small intestine has the assigned task of churning and mixing nutritive elements with digestive juices. This permits the breakdown of fats, protein, and carbohydrates into their smallest components for assimilation into the body. Contraction and relaxation of these intestinal wall muscles are what propel raw materials on their way to the next digestive station to face the action of various hormones and enzymes. Quite likely, the many intestinal glands share in the general problem of fibromyalgia and, along with the muscles, prove inadequate for an ideal digestive sequence. Constipation and diarrhea are like changing traffic signals for the stop and go prompting of the digestive and eliminative processes. As you would imagine, this causes serious malfunction in the entire gastrointestinal tract, certainly enough to produce all of the symptoms of irritable bowel syndrome.

Foods are processed, broken down, and absorbed mainly in the small intestine. The colon lies downstream and also serves many functions. Its muscles and glands are also affected in fibromyalgia and therefore contribute more than just mucus to the irritable bowel syndrome. Bacteria have taken up a permanent abode in the colon, whereas the small intestine is normally free of them. These organisms use our food residues for their metabolic needs and, in the process, provide us with certain benefits. As much as twenty percent of ingested carbohydrates reach the large intestine undigested. These carbohydrates are the main source of nutrition for the bacteria. Unfortunately, they greatly add to our gas when they ferment sugar and starch residues. Gas can cause repetitive, sharp stabs of pain in the small intestine, but it does not linger there. It is propelled along and quickly expelled into the much larger collecting areas of the colon. The contractions of the colon's more forceful muscles direct the digestive remnants toward the rectum for elimination. Gas is moved downstream and distends the colon wherever it temporarily accumulates. Large pockets collect in certain areas, since air rises to the highest point.

Typical sites for pain are the lower right abdomen, where gas first arrives from the small intestine. As pressure builds in that area, the gas is driven to the upper right abdomen, at the edge of the liver. Most distressing, however, is the pain produced in the left upper abdomen, the highest point in the colon just under the heart. When it is distended, that location can shoot sharp stabs of pain into the chest in front of the heart. When the intestinal muscles contract, the results are a bit like grabbing a long, sausage-like balloon in the middle. The gas squeezes in both directions but, as soon as one end lets go, it gushes back to the center site. In the gassy fibromyalgic, this is not a very effective means of transport, and patients suffer repeated pains from the shifting gas.

Gas adds to the problem in other ways. It is made up of the usual components found in air, but some of them are present in different concentrations. Stools inside the body exposed to the effects of air are further dried and hardened. Constipation is made worse, and the cement-like stools further irritate the sigmoid colon. This leads to more spasms, hemorrhoids, fissures, and bleeding, as we discussed above. The hard stool plugs up the rectal area and acts like a dam against the elimination of gas; as a result, more bloating and drying occur. This in turn adds greatly to the existing discomfort and can cause nausea. Patients are miserable and yearn for "comfort foods," the easily digested sugars and starches. Our statistics show that sixty percent of our fibromyalgics begin craving sweets in their unsuccessful attempt to make energy, as we discussed in another chapter. Carbohydrates feed the bacteria that make more gas and intensify the discomfort of the irritable bowel syndrome. Worse, they also promote the tendency toward hypoglycemia or increase its symptoms greatly if the condition already exists.

As we have already described, the repetitive release of insulin increases carbohydrate conversion to fat in the liver. Using an arbitrary weight gain of twenty pounds as a measure of obesity, we found that thirty-five percent of our fibromyalgics have gained that amount, and often much more, during the course of their illness. Obesity, in turn, adds all of its ill effects to the endocrine system, muscles, joints, and digestion, with loss of energy and self-esteem. In susceptible people, this is all that is necessary to produce insulin insensitivity and, ultimately, diabetes. Although I do not plan to discuss these dangers in further detail, they are genuine threats to health.

> I was never diagnosed with IBS until we arrived at the FMS and HG [hypoglycemia] diagnosis. Everything was a mystery. I had been plagued all my life with inexplicable stomach and intestinal pains, gas and bloating, alternating diarrhea and constipation. The most common medical advice was to "relax" and take antacids. I have been on the hypoglycemia diet, alternating between strict and liberal versions, for almost a year. I have managed to completely eliminate the IBS symptoms after a month on the strict diet.
> —*G.W., Los Angeles*

Another common diagnostic pitfall is the dull, aching pain that can arise from the muscles of the abdominal wall. What frequently occurs is that the physician diligently completes his or her studies of the problem and ends up with normal findings. The pain is usually ascribed to the IBS as just another symptom of that disease. The internal pain of IBS, which is due to cramping or gas pressure, is quite different from the surface aching that arises from spasm in the abdominal wall muscles. These muscle contractions are no different from the ones that occur throughout the rest of the body. I try to distinguish this particular type of aching during my examination by asking patients to lie down and raise their heads off the pillow. This tenses the abdominal muscle quite well, and I can feel the difference in tension by comparing one side to the other. The tense parts of these muscles are identical to the swollen and contracted areas I find in any other fibromyalgic muscle.

A frequently overlooked cause of abdominal pain is due to involvement of the inguinal ligaments. These double, parallel cords are present on each side of the groin, and they run from the pelvic bone in front of the hip to the pubic bone. The abdominal muscles actually form the ligament as they curl around each other and make the rope-like structure that attaches and secures them. They are almost always involved in fibromyalgia and are easily felt as swollen areas in the ligament, more toward the outside portions. When the ligaments are involved, they create a steady pull on the attached muscles and put them into spasm, usually higher up in the abdomen. This tensing action can cause pain on the underside of the rib margins, where the muscles attach.

Origins of Abdominal Pain

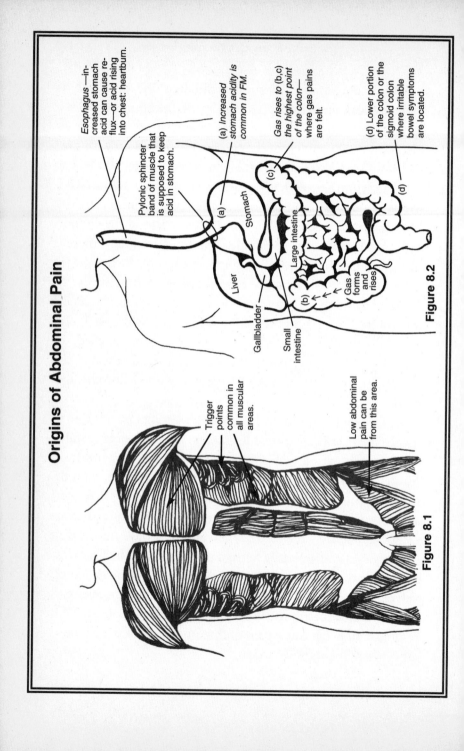

Figure 8.2

Esophagus —increased stomach acid can cause reflux—or acid rising into chest: heartburn.

Pylonic sphincter band of muscle that is supposed to keep acid in stomach.

(a) *Increased stomach acidity is common in FM.*

Gas rises to (b,c) the highest point of the colon—where gas pains are felt.

(d) Lower portion of the colon or the sigmoid colon where irritable bowel symptoms are located.

Liver

Gallbladder

Stomach

Large intestine

Small intestine

Gas forms and rises

(a)

(b)

(c)

(d)

Figure 8.1

Trigger points common in all muscular areas.

Low abdominal pain can be from this area.

When the lower part of the large intestine, the sigmoid colon, causes painful spasms, various medications are prescribed. Some of these do reduce symptoms. However, patients also seek over-the-counter products such as a variety of antacids, cathartics, and gas-reducing agents that are often worthless since they are directed to the wrong purpose. However, sometimes individuals simply add these to their prescription drugs in a "shotgun" approach. Costs rise as patients pile one gastrointestinal drug on top of another. Adding this fistful of pills to those they already use for sleep, nervousness, depression, and pain will certainly make their pharmacist's monthly car payments but also increases chances for unfavorable drug interactions. More often than not, patients ingest some drugs that actually make their constipation worse. Among these are the narcotic derivatives of codeine, muscle relaxants such as Flexeril and Soma, and most of the antidepressants that are so freely given. Although some patients use laxatives regularly, they should be warned that these could be habit-forming. Patients usually dread eliminating even one of their medications since they consider them all an integral part of their drug armamentarium. Any omission leads to fear and the risk that things might be even slightly worse without it. Their concern is well founded in their knowledge that they have no remaining emotional or physical reserves. They cannot contemplate, however briefly, how they would cope with even one more aggravation. Pharmaceutical companies may make many gastrointestinal "Band-Aids" but I prefer to treat the cause of an illness and only secondarily its symptoms. The story below is typical:

For the last ten years or so I have been diagnosed with everything from colitis to food allergies to systemic candida infection because I have had so much trouble with diarrhea. Sometimes I would go for days with no bowel function and then out of the blue I'd have diarrhea. . . . I had constant painful intestinal gas that was very embarrassing because I could not control it. I was treated for colitis and then sprue or gluten intolerance. Neither of those treatments helped. Next, an allergist diagnosed me with intestinal yeast infections from antibiotics. He said I had developed food allergies from the yeast and put me on an antifungal drug called nystatin. That helped a little. The next doctor . . . did a two-year series of European allergy shots and gave me an even stronger drug for the yeast. [He] had me injecting myself with allergy shots two to three times a week and taking doses and potions of various things by mouth four times a day. My diet was very restricted, and my weight fell from 118 to 98 pounds. The doctor had me on a high-carbohydrate diet in a failed attempt at weight gain.

In desperation and prayer I turned to the Internet and found Dr. St. Amand's information. After comparing his description of hypoglycemia and IBS to my symptoms, I hoped I had found an answer. I dropped Dr. St. Amand and Claudia an e-mail. Dr. St. Amand assured me I was on the right track. Claudia helped me get started on the diet and told me what to do in the stormy early weeks, as my body fought to adjust to the new fuel. She promised after the first six weeks things would settle down. They did. The gas and diarrhea and other symptoms are gone now as long as I stay on the diet. . . . The good news is I can now eat anything on the HG diet and

not have diarrhea or gas. I no longer look like a starved
waif, having put on 14 pounds as well.
—*Gretchen, South Carolina*

Patients with irritable bowel syndrome usually suffer as
deeply in their relationships as do those with vulvodynia and
bladder dysfunction. All three of these conditions isolate the
individual because of the personal nature of the affected areas.
Many times, people suffer in silence, not knowing how to explain their illness to others. They tend to keep to themselves and
avoid discussing their problems, even at home and certainly in
the workplace. Several self-help groups, support groups, and
information services exist. We have listed some of these in the
Resources section in the back of this book.

🐚 TREATMENT

So how do we treat this irritable bowel syndrome? These are
the simplest paragraphs in this entire chapter. Begin with the
elimination of sugars and complex carbohydrates. You will
find the proper diet outlined in the hypoglycemia chapter.
The diet is the same as for hypoglycemia. These dietary restrictions will be temporary for most of you. You will quickly
eliminate some symptoms with the diet alone. Once you feel
better, add your favorite foods one at a time and back off when
the symptoms recur, trusting this as an indication that you've
added too much, too often. This hunt-and-peck system is really the only way to learn how frequently you can tolerate "ju-
dicious" cheating. The premenstrual week is the most delicate
time for such testing. It is the riskiest week of the month for
resurrecting adverse effects. In time, you will learn what you

need to restrict on a permanent basis, if anything. You will develop your own, personal program.

The remaining treatment format is equally simple. The steps to be followed are clearly defined in the chapter dealing with guaifenesin treatment, Chapter 6. I will summarize them briefly here. Basically, you will have to find your personal dosage with the help of your doctor and some of your own observations. At the same time, you must eliminate the blocking effects of salicylates—that is your job. You've probably realized that each of the preceding chapters on fibromyalgia, fibroglycemia, genitourinary syndrome, and now this one on irritable bowel syndrome are actually an artificial division made to simplify our discussions. This entire book has been written for one purpose only: purging fibromyalgia and controlling the hypoglycemia that often accompanies it. Over the years, many of you already suspected that this network of symptoms and these so-called syndromes were all connected, long before you picked up this book. Luckily, we are dealing with at most only the two interlocking diseases of fibromyalgia and hypoglycemia, and we strongly advocate only one medication and one diet to control all the symptoms of both conditions.

WARNING

Irritable bowel syndrome and fibromyalgia do not cause a high fever or severe pain that are persistent. If you are experiencing these symptoms, with or without nausea, diarrhea, or constipation, see a doctor to rule out more dangerous conditions such as appendicitis or diverticulitis.

Chapter 9

The Brain Symptoms: Chronic Fatigue,
Fibrofog, Fibrofrustration

For me personally, depression, anxiety, and severe cognitive problems were my major FMS symptoms before going into full body
pain. I was put on almost every antidepressant in the book. The
doctors focused on my emotional symptoms, which led them to
overlook the physical FMS symptoms I had been exhibiting for
years. . . . After 54 doctors from up and down the eastern
seaboard, it took one last desperate trip to the Mayo Clinic for diagnosis. . . . Before guai I was on many medications, which I felt
were making me feel worse. After finding Dr. St. Amand's material, I realized I was not losing my mind but had the symptoms of
FMS. I was able to understand why I had become like I did and
view the depression as a symptom that I could now help. . . . In
less than two months, I was off all my medication except thyroid
and hormone replacement therapy.

—*Jayne W., Tarpon Springs, FL*

The cerebral, or brain, cycles of fibromyalgia have entered
medical literature somewhat late in the game, and mostly
through the back door. Recent books written by fibromyalgics,
such as Doctor Devin Starlanyl, devote entire chapters to the
toll the disease has taken on her cognitive abilities. The original spate of papers written in the 1980s by the experts busy

defining fibromyalgia (Doctors Smythe, Bennett, Goldenberg, Yunus, Wolfe, and others) were mostly about tender or trigger points, sleep disturbances, and comparative studies of pain medications. In the beginning, fibromyalgia was viewed as a physical pain syndrome. Although this was a pleasant change for patients who had been told too often their symptoms were all in their head, it did little to help them understand that their fatigue and cognitive impairments were a normal part of their illness. A debate began as researchers desperately sought an answer to the question: Is depression the cause or the effect of fibromyalgia? It was eventually determined by large, controlled studies that fibromyalgics were no more nor less depressed than any other group of patients who lived in chronic pain.

"Fibromyalgia was often considered to be a manifestation of hysteria and was equated with psychogenic rheumatism in the 1950s and '60s. However, with recent controlled studies it became evident that patients with this syndrome had uniform, stable and reproducible symptoms and signs rather than the bizarre and changeable symptoms of hysteria."[23]

The result of these studies was that, by and large, depression and an impaired ability to function mentally are now recognized as part of fibromyalgia. Nearly all doctors today realize that fibromyalgia is not a psychological illness. A few doctors, usually in private practice, stubbornly continue to believe so. They will point out that antidepressants work in treating the disease, not realizing that this is far from a general rule. Research scientists now believe that reason for this pharmacological overlap is that pain and depression may share some of the same receptors, and a medication that has effects on one can logically be expected to have some effect on the other.

I lose trains of thought and action, blank out frequently for brief periods, ride emotional waves of hope and despair, struggle to make my brain function with clarity, suffer memory loss (sometimes total, sometimes recoverable with help), cannot make sense of small print and complex reading, cannot keep my place in following a recipe or shopping list, struggle with almost total frustration trying to organize information/tools/tasks, do not take in what I am reading or almost instantly forget what I have just read, have to proofread what I write several times, and still miss errors, am easily distracted and so on. . . . Certainly stress, overdoing it, too many distractions, and fatigue increase my mental disabilities, just as they increase all of my other FMS symptoms.

—Virginia, Texas

There is no doubt whatsoever to those who have the disease that "brain cycles" exist in fibromyalgia. Unfortunately, the mechanism that causes them remains obscure. Brain cycles coincide with pain cycles, and so can last for a few hours, a few weeks, or for months. When a patient's pain level diminishes, these other symptoms do too. We have found that as guaifenesin treatment reverses the physical pain of fibromyalgia, the cognitive symptoms clear as well.

These cognitive problems include some of the most debilitating symptoms of FMS. They are the equal of pain cycles in their negative impact on quality of life, and many patients consider them worse. Patients suffer from the sensation of a scattered mind, waves of depression, fatigue, irritability, impaired memory and concentration, apathy, insomnia, nonrestorative sleep, nervousness, and a sensation that the brain is not connected to the body. The misery of these symptoms is exacerbated by the fact that patients have difficulty expressing themselves.

❦ CHRONIC FATIGUE SYNDROME: FIBROFATIGUE

> My biggest symptoms are fatigue and exhaustion. It has not been unusual to go to the store and be there for a bit and suddenly feel like a big syringe sucked out all my energy. I would immediately have to sit down or go to the car and lie down. When I had a job sometimes I would close my office and lie down. Sometimes I can feel it coming on but other times suddenly I will just become weak. I don't have a lot of pain like the kind I've heard others describe. For that I am thankful, because I can manage with OTC pain medications. My next set of symptoms come and go but do hamper my life quite a bit. Brain fog, nausea (at times to the point of throwing up), dizziness, and rare panic attacks.
>
> *—Heather Lock, Texas*

Forty years ago when I began working with the disease that was to eventually be named fibromyalgia, I noted that while patients had many symptoms in common, there was also a great individual variability. Some had intense pain all over, some complained of continuous numbing fatigue. Most were in pain *and* tired. Examination revealed that they all had very real physical findings—palpable lumps and bumps in muscles and tendons. Detailed histories established that they had many more symptoms in common than it initially seemed, enough to prove to me that I was dealing with one disease that encompassed a spectrum of symptoms.

Now, at last, in well-detailed medical papers, the symptom overlap between fibromyalgia and chronic fatigue has been made obvious. Most physicians now believe they are the same malady. I have treated thousands of patients, and I can state that I have never seen a case of pure chronic fatigue syndrome. When a careful history is taken, and a body map is made, all of the symptoms and findings meet the criteria for fibromyalgia. It is my experience that when patients have extremely high pain thresholds, fatigue is their dominant complaint. Careful questioning can elicit the symptoms of irritable bowel, bladder or vulvar pain as well as musculoskeletal complaints that seem mild to patients when compared to their fatigue and cognitive dysfunction. They have the same palpable changes in their muscles, tendons, and ligaments. The worst "map" I ever made of a patient was of a woman who said she had zero pain, only mild stiffness—she also had dental work and her babies without anesthetics. We have treated these so-called chronic fatigue syndrome patients with guaifenesin and have had the same success as with those who complain primarily of pain.

In fibromyalgia, fatigue often goes hand in hand with sleeplessness. Even in healthy people, lack of sleep causes impaired mental function. Fibromyalgics cannot sleep well and awaken frequently throughout the night, especially during their pain cycles. Patients are tempted to increase the dosage of their sleeping medications, in the hope that deeper sleep will clear the mental fogginess. Since sleep deprivation does not cause fibromyalgia, sleep alone will not make the brain symptoms go away. It should be remembered that sleep medications cause slower mental connections the next day, even in healthy patients. Taking them when fatigued can initiate a vicious circle in which mental clarity suffers even more.

> Exhaustion has always been a major problem for me. Especially the past six months or so. I've been in the habit of taking some form of natural energy boosters (ginseng, guarana, etc.) for at least the past 10 years. Since I'm on guaifenesin, I can't do that anymore, so I'm now having a very hard time making it through each day. Sometimes I think I feel good, and then go to the grocery store, and after five minutes feel like I have walked five miles. Sometimes I have to rest my head on my desk or my hands, and take a little "nap" at work. I have a high tolerance for pain, but also for medications. My body just laughs at OTC stuff. I even have to take double what most people do for prescription drugs, so I mostly just have to deal with the pain on my own, unless it is so bad I can't walk, write, etc. I think exhaustion is a big part of FMS, and that we all have to endure it. For me it is always there, even when the pain isn't.

> *Progress report—a few months later:*

> As an update, I am so much better it's unreal. I'm on 600 mg/day of guaifenesin now, am working 40 [or more] hours a week, and even take the stairs at work! I still have a bad day now and then (one or two a month), but my progress is so amazing, my doctor has started other patients he has with fibromyalgia on what he calls "the Tisdale Therapy." He says I'm his poster

child for fibromyalgia. But between the guai and changing all my medications around (I finally got off Prozac after 10 years!), I've lost the bluish color in my hands, I don't sweat all the time now, and overall, I feel pretty normal. My doctor says he's amazed at the difference from when I walked into his office last April.

—*Sherry L., Atlanta, GA*

Fatigue in fibromyalgia may be omnipresent, but in a flare, patients become so exhausted that they cannot concentrate on even simple cognitive activities. They often find that a nap is helpful, even a short one. Most patients do not have trouble falling asleep; in fact they commonly collapse from exhaustion early in the evening. In the morning patients wake up unrefreshed and feeling as if they have been run over by a truck, even after ten or more hours in bed.

Guaifenesin will reverse the fatigue and insomnia cycles of fibromyalgia. Patients will notice fewer days of exhaustion and will eventually be rewarded with a high-energy day that will give them encouragement to continue. These first days with abundant energy are dramatic, and patients never forget them.

❦ FIBROFOG AND FIBROFRUSTRATION

These bad periods creep up. You think you are handling everything and then the pain starts to increase and suddenly you are in a panic. . . . When the pain starts, I think I can still continue doing what I have been doing. What creeps up on me is the brain confusion. I get so frustrated trying to sort out the simplest things, until I give up and then I get depressed.

How do I handle it? Recognizing it for what it is comes first. Then I just have to let go of everything I don't have to do, and keep things very simple, rest a lot, baby myself. Get a massage, physical therapy, pool therapy for pain, or take whatever medications help.

It is interesting for me to watch this cycle towards depression and see how it is based on brain dysfunction and expectations. The mood swings go with the cycling too. . . . You can't expect too much of yourself when you don't feel well. Your brain is just trying to tell you that.

—*L.N., Massachusetts*

Physicians who treat fibromyalgics know that almost every patient has said at one time or another: "I can stand the pain, but I need my brain." These are the patients who suffer severely from *fibrofog*. Patients can best describe a "brain fog" as if their brains were in a deep overcast which keeps them from interacting with their own body and being responsive to the rest of the world. Their short-term memory is bad; they cannot remember things they have just been told. This and the fact that their sense of direction is disrupted cause patients to get lost even in places they know very well. They often forget what they are doing or saying in the middle of a task. Reasoning and deduction range from difficult to impossible, depending on the severity of a cycle. Patients cannot read because they cannot absorb the material, follow a plot, or remember the names of characters. Common also is an inability to spell words or recognize if they are written correctly. More than one patient has told me that when fibrofog is bad, they can't even use a dictionary—they have no idea about the sequence of letters or even the alphabet.

Patients cannot remember where they left things, cannot "see things" even when they are looking directly at them, or remember what they are looking for. They completely forget appointments and things they are supposed to do, and cannot remember whether or not they have paid their bills. Fibrofrustration, caused by the inability to count on one's own brain, is demoralizing and increases a patient's irritability, nervousness, anxiety, and sense of isolation.

During these brain cycles, patients become oversensitive to noise, bright lights, smells, and other external stimuli. Ordinary sounds from television may cause severe discomfort. For others, the noise from fluorescent lights is intolerable. Most patients describe sensitivity to smells to some degree. These various stimuli increase mental symptoms and add to anxiety and frustration, and can heighten physical symptoms such as headaches or nausea. It is not surprising that these symptom combinations have led some doctors to think of fibromyalgia as a sensitivity syndrome that is caused by exposure to contaminants in our environment. This has induced many physicians to specialize in environmental medicine. In our experience, when a patient feels well, these symptoms usually recede along with the others.

It is important for patients to learn coping skills when dealing with fibrofog. The less fibrofrustration they experience, the more bearable will be these impaired cognitive cycles. The underlying fear of forgetting something important, of not being able to count on one's memory, is a great stress that amplifies the intensity of other symptoms.

- Practice being methodical, so that it becomes second nature. Develop simple habits. Train yourself to put things in the same place every time. For example, put your car keys on a peg by the door. If you always put them there, eventually you will do it without thinking about it. It will become a habit. No matter how exhausted you are, every time you come into the house, hang your keys on the same peg. Mail box keys, glasses, unpaid bills, mail to be answered, shopping lists—these should all have a special, well-marked place.

- Put up a big calendar in a prominent place, such as on your refrigerator. Write down every appointment the minute you make it. Every morning and every night check this calendar. Do it at two specific times: just before you go to bed and when you have morning coffee. If you're afraid you'll forget something during the day, hang a note up where you are sure to see it.

- Make a list of what you have to do. Then train yourself to check the list routinely several times a day. When you get up in the morning, check your list. When you complete a task, cross it off right away, in case you cannot remember later whether or not you've done it. Never leave the house without checking your list of things to do. When you go out, take a copy with you if you have the habit of forgetting one of your errands.

- Keep a pad and a pen near the phone and make sure you leave them there. Don't walk off with them. When you take a message, write it down. Sometimes when the fog is very bad you may want to make notes while you are talking. You may even need to do this to remember to whom you were speaking. Keep the notes concise, so that you can figure them out later.

- Post notes. Many patients have told me they cannot imagine what they did before Post-its, those little papers with a sticky part. Some hang up notes reminding them to turn off lights, lock doors, water their plants, and remember shopping lists, children's school schedules, or athletic practices. Sometimes you will want to post notes in other places, such as on the dashboard of your car.

- Make lists to take to your appointments. If you have a meeting with your child's teacher, boss, repairmen, or a client, make a list of pertinent things. Make one to take with you when you go to the doctor. There is nothing more frustrating for doctor and patient when a patient walks out of the appointment room and suddenly remembers a question she forgot to ask. During an appointment, make notes if you think you will forget answers or facts. You should do the same at your children's schools and even when making arrangements with family and friends.

- If you're in a severe fibrofog, limit your driving. Run one errand at a time. Save complicated ones for when you are feeling better. If you drive, turn off the radio. This will help you concentrate on driving. Instruct your passengers and children to keep quiet, and insist on it. If your children are noisy and this confuses or distracts you, pull over and explain the situation to them. Use surface streets whenever possible. Missing freeway exits and going far out of your way can certainly increase fibrofrustration.

- At home and at work, decrease your sensory input. Many patients find they absolutely cannot function with background noises. For some reason they lose the ability to tune them out or keep them in the background. Turn off music while working. Even the most soothing music can make some of you feel overloaded in a cycle. Filter out noise by closing the doors of the room where you are working to let you concentrate in silence.

- Start working on projects early. Plan on your work taking twice as long as it usually does. Your ability to absorb information is impaired. If work is impossible, give it up and try later. Sometimes you will have no alternative but to take a break from a frustrating task.

🐚 MOOD SWINGS (FIBROFLUX)

A normal but horrifying part of brain cycling are mood swings. For the most part, patients are acutely aware of them but feel powerless to exercise control. Anger, frustration, fear, depression, and self-pity can come and go in the matter of minutes with great intensity. Patients will notice that they cry easily and become frustrated and angry at the slightest provocation.

The reason for these mood swings, again, is unclear. Some doctors have speculated fluctuating or abnormal hormone levels; others believe the fault may lie somehow with neurotransmitters. Dr. Devin Starlanyl has devised the name "fibroflux" for these unpleasant symptoms.

Most important of all is to recognize that all these cognitive impairments and emotional overreactions are a normal part of fibromyalgia experienced to some degree by those who suffer from the disease. Be patient and understanding with yourself. Remember to laugh when your fibrofog has caused you to do something funny. Laughter is one medicine that everyone agrees helps with all chronic diseases, including fibromyalgia.

Chapter 10

Other Symptoms

With entire chapters in this book devoted to genitourinary syndrome, gastrointestinal or irritable bowel syndrome, and fibrofog, you may think that we have covered every possible aspect of FMS. However, in our treatment of this illness, we have discovered even more body systems that are affected and also deserve to be explored. In some patients, for example, FMS can affect the skin, nails, hair, and other tissues—these disturbances form their own niche but should not be overlooked in any comprehensive discussion of fibromyalgia.

SKIN

> I have had this consistently since I got sick; my first symptoms being fatigue, itching rashes, and hives. I have been a notorious complainer about pins and needles, tingling, and painful burning of the skin. The itching intensified when I started the guai in Novem-

ber 1996. I used to use Benadryl almost every night for this. I also tried Caladryl, Benadryl cream, cortisone cream, etc. I have found several things that help: (1) Dry brushing with a bath brush before a shower. (2) Using a bath brush in a bath with Epsom salts, sea salts, and baking soda (1 cup each). Take a shower afterwards to wash off the salt. (3) Lac-Hydrin or Aquaphor lotion. (4) Benadryl or prescription medications for itching or sleep at night. It has started to get better for me after a year and three months on guai.

—*Heather Lock, Texas*

The skin is the largest of the body's organs and is deeply affected by fibromyalgia. We have seen all types of rashes, from eczema to acne, seborrhea, hives, tiny dry bumps, and small blistered patches of skin. Nails and hair are commonly of poor quality.

A scientific paper recently reported the infiltration of *immunoglobulin G* and the breaking of *mast cells* deep in the skin tissue of people with FMS. These mast cells release histamine, often the perpetrator of itching and funny rashes, mainly hives. Immunoglobulin G attests to the body's perception of something foreign or at least annoying to tissues.[24]

Other studies show that fibromyalgics often have a higher than normal level of *histamines.* The body releases these when it perceives danger—either physically, as a result of an injury, or when threatened from exposure to a foreign protein. High histamine levels result in swelling and the common allergy symptoms such as itchy, watery eyes, and a runny nose.

It is only in recent years that we have realized the extent of skin involvement in fibromyalgia. We have regularly heard patients describe tingling sensations, most commonly in the fingers and toes, but also in scattered areas such as the face and lips. All kinds of other, weird sensations are described. Crawling feelings anywhere on the skin used to make me try to brush off an insect that was never there. Burning can be felt anywhere on the surface of the body, commonly on the back of the neck. It is common for fibromyalgics to cut the tags out of their clothes because of this sensation. The intensity of this burning can also be extreme. When it affected the soles of my feet, I would have to kick them out from under the covers at night.

Patients often describe intense itching. It can occur anywhere, and patients say it sometimes comes on so strongly that they feel it will never stop. Universally, the itching appears to be worse at night. The warmth generated under the blankets seems to set it off, and often the itching seems more widespread then than at any other time. In my own case, when the itching began in the evening, I knew I was in for a bad night's sleep. The rest of my fibromyalgia symptoms were likely to join in.

Over the years, our patients have described a multitude of rashes. Isolated or generalized hives are among the most common. One woman, a flight attendant, was the first to show me how intensely this could affect a person. Long before she came to me, she had times when a strange type of giant hives appeared that oddly involved only her face and neck. Redness and an unusual amount of swelling always accompanied them. She told me that in these attacks she looked "like a gargoyle." The one time I saw her with them I had to compliment her on the accuracy of her description. On her hives days, she had to call in sick and cancel her flights.

She was an interesting woman, both as a person, and medically speaking. She had undergone extensive testing for allergies and *autoimmune diseases.* When I first began treating her, I never for a moment thought that there was a connection between her hives and her fibromyalgia. When she began treatment, the mystery gradually unraveled. It was not long before she realized that her hives appeared only when she was in a pain cycle. She never had hives when she was feeling well. As you would expect from my story, she is now almost totally free of her fibromyalgia, and in her rare and mild reversal cycles she no longer has hives.

This is not to say that I didn't know about other rashes and *their* relationship to fibromyalgia. Most patients described dry patches of skin that had scaling and itching in various places on their bodies. If these patches were extensive or annoying enough, patients had already consulted dermatologists or their family doctors, who routinely diagnosed their condition as *eczema,* or some other skin condition. The worst case of *neurodermatitis* I have ever seen was on a young attorney. His face and hands were his main problem, since clients could readily see these areas of involvement. He had stopped offering his handshake because of his scaling, cracking hands. His muscular aches and pains were minimal but he did have some cognitive difficulties and fatigue. Examination confirmed his diagnosis with the telltale lumps and bumps of fibromyalgia. His rash initially became worse with each reverse cycle, and has now cleared completely.

My own patches of *seborrheic dermatitis* tormented me with raw, burning sensations. I also had eruptions of tiny blisters that appeared mainly between my fingers. My patients complained of these as well, some with the same blisters in other areas of their bodies. Patients with psoriasis observed that their rash became much worse during attacks of fibromyalgia. I spoke to a support group one night and found it difficult to take my eyes off one woman's face. Her skin was almost a magenta color. She later became my patient, and she and her husband noticed that her amazing color came only with attacks. She is now symptom-free and says she doesn't miss her strange patina. Flushes and redness experienced by patients, especially just before the onset of pain cycles, are obviously not from the skin itself but rather from the underlying blood vessels that suddenly dilate. The skin can also display *dermatographia.* In this condition, one can use a fingernail or blunt instrument, and literally write on the patient's skin. The result is redness and a slight swelling as the dermal capillaries that reproduce the written inscriptions visibly indicate to us. We don't know the effect of fibromyalgia on the walls of capillaries, but these symptoms are extremely common. These symptoms may all be related to the fact that the release of histamines is known to cause an increase in the permeability of the capillaries.

> I have never had the severe itching sensation that some fibromyalgics describe. I feel *pain.* It feels like a burn *inside* my skin. When I'm touched, it feels like that burning skin is being scraped. I have had itching symptoms with a rash. No apparent cause, and it eventually went away after about a week. No skin medications helped these conditions.
>
> —*J.M., Texas*

🐚 FINGERNAILS

The chipping and breaking of fingernails is so common that I question all my patients about it when I take their medical history during their initial visit. It is even common for women to tell me that the quality of their fingernails is so poor that they cannot wear acrylic nails because their own nails are too weak to support them. I also hear of nails that peel like a sheet of mica, nails that bend backwards easily, and nails that break too easily, causing repeated hangnails. The cuticles are even affected. They often thicken, then split and tear. In most patients, nail growth seems normal, but all of a sudden, for no apparent reason, all the nails break at once. This phenomenon is easily understood if one thinks of the nail as having concentric rings, like a tree. During the cycles of fibromyalgia, when the temporary flood of our abnormality is in the bloodstream, deposits of brittle calcium phosphate are laid down at the nail root. This occurs whether the disease is in its developmental stages or reversal cycles. Eight to nine months later, the faulty part of the nail that was formed during these cycles reaches the tip and chips or breaks off. When patients are first hit with FMS, the nails grow fairly well because they have alternating good layers with bad ones. In long-standing fibromyalgia, the nails develop no good layers and they remain broken all the time.

🐚 HAIR

You will notice [after beginning guaifenesin] your hair is getting back to normal, actually better. Mine used to be dry, but got to where I could go a few days before I had to wash it (when I was sick, I didn't wash it for three days and it wasn't greasy). My hair is very healthy now. Just give it some time. I am taking 3600 mg of guaifenesin a day, and have been totally pain free for about three months.

—*M.B.F.*

In fibromyalgics, the hair is often defective and has a poor quality, splitting ends, and slow growth. These tissues are actually outgrowths of the skin—the dermis. As a general rule, patients seem to notice some hair loss at about the fourth or fifth month of successful reversal with guaifenesin. When they first notice this, it always frightens them, and usually generates a phone call. I have given up referring patients to dermatologists as I used to. Numerous work-ups produced no results. Hairdressers have turned out to be my best allies since they explain to their clients that a certain amount of hair loss is normal. Patients soon find new growth that is much improved in quality.

❧ OTHER TISSUES

I could always tell when my younger son, Sean, was in a cycle, although he did not complain much of pain. When I would wake him up for school in the mornings, his eyes would be almost glued shut with gooky stuff. I would have to put a wet washcloth over his eyes and let it sit there for a while to soak this off. The clumps in his eyelashes were stiff and incredibly hard to get out. Those were the days when he would wake up irritable and tired, and have the most trouble in school.

—*C.C., La Jolla, CA*

Most fibromyalgics also have problems with the so-called inner skin, the mucosa that lines our moist tissues. The inner eyelids and eyes themselves frequently itch, redden, and release mucus. In the daytime, this is wiped away unconsciously. When it occurs at night, it dries by morning and forms sand in the corners of the eye. Patients who wear contact lenses find that during cycles they are often blurry, and when taken out, appear covered with a film. During the day, one's eyes can itch and constantly feel irritated or strained. Bright lights and television or computer screens can make this sensation worse. Patients find that lying down in a darkened room with a cool cloth over their eyes can ease this feeling.

In addition to the eyes, the mucosa around the mouth can also be affected. For some patients, it is common to wake up with a rash around the mouth, especially in the corners. This rash is apparently caused by the exposure of the skin to the patient's own saliva. This irritating and acidy saliva may also be the reason for the burned, scalded, and metallic tastes patients often complain about.

Even more mucosal tissues are also affected by fibromyalgia. The lining of the nose, bronchial tubes, vagina, and rectum all produce mucus that may be acidic and irritating. Many women describe the vulvar skin and the skin on the inner thighs looking like it has been chemically burned. Their partners may also have this same burn in the pubic area following intercourse. We can only guess about the effects on the mucosa of the stomach and small intestine and how this contributes to the irritable bowel syndrome.

> I just got over the itching. It lasted for three weeks. All the Benadryl and prescriptions for itching didn't help it much at all. What helped me was just plain Tylenol or Advil. Heat seemed to make it worse but ice did help. I was also given a prescription for a lotion to use that would keep the skin from looking too bad from all of the scratching. It was Aquaphor ointment. After my itching was finally over, I did go into a pain cycle and am now coming out of it. In fact today I feel pretty good. Yay Guai!
>
> *—Katy, Arkansas*

The dermal symptoms of fibromyalgia are frequently a great concern to patients. More than any other complex of symptoms, they affect one's outward appearance. For fibromyalgics who are already feeling unattractive and tired, the addition of rashes and hives or pimples can be demoralizing. It is a great comfort to patients, both mentally and physically, when their skin returns to normal with guaifenesin.

❦ BONES: FIBROMYALGIA AND OSTEOARTHRITIS

Fibromyalgia is only the beginning of a long, miserable process which, I believe, leads ultimately to osteoarthritis. This is not the crippling kind of arthritis that causes severe deformities, though it can certainly damage joints to the point of requiring knee or hip replacements. Most people accept aches and stiffness as a normal part of growing older, so osteoarthritis is generally thought of as "the wear and tear arthritis" of the elderly.

When we examine our patients' older family members who have been diagnosed with osteoarthritis, they pour out symptoms that say to us that they began long ago as fibromyalgics. The difference is that now joint pains are their predominant symptoms, and their X rays show the spurs and other destructive changes we call "*osteo*" (from *os*, the Latin word for bone) arthritis. I am not alluding here to a joint that has been damaged in an accident. This is traumatic arthritis, and symptoms from this are limited to the areas that suffered the injury.

Why are joints the last area of the body to suffer from fibromyalgia? It is always striking to me how the body of a fibromyalgic manages to avoid damage to its most essential organs. There is never cell death or muscular wasting (atrophy), and no nerve damage with fibromyalgia. The kidneys perform normally except for the small error my theory proposes. The liver remains normal and the heart continues to beat. The brain still directs traffic, albeit erratically in the presence of fibrofog. Cuts still heal. The body remains capable of fighting disease.

But we know that under the influence of the genetic abnormality that causes fibromyalgia, eventually something has to give. It seems logical that the body is willing and able to sacrifice less crucial functions and anatomical sites in order to protect the most important ones. There even seems to be a roughly beneficial sequence as the disease first hits the areas that will cause the least loss of function. Bones have likely done their utmost, early on, right from birth, as powerful and effective buffers. The brain, intestine, and urinary tract suffer off and on, and do their part in stashing the excess incoming phosphate and calcium. Tendons and ligaments seem safe structures to accept abnormal stores. Even with this excess, they can continue to do their jobs reasonably well since they are only required to make limited stretches. Logically, then, muscles are next in the reception line. It is at this point when patients most commonly present themselves to doctors complaining of pain and fatigue.

As the disease process continues, a truce can be called in any given tissue, but only by greatly slowing its production of ATP. At this point equilibrium must be reached to prevent cell death (apoptosis). This is the damage control mechanism available for each area, and it is this limitation in forming ATP that saves the cell from destruction. Reduced energy availability allows the cell to survive and not to work until it destroys itself. Then the fibromyalgic process must move on to find another available area for tucking away the excess ions.

When the muscles cannot accept any more, the joints are recruited and become the ultimate tuckable site for this progressive retention of excess phosphate and its fellow traveler, calcium. Joints display an inexhaustible capacity and continue to accept deposits throughout the rest of the fibromyalgic's life. Crystals actually form in these areas, whereas in other tissues, calcium and phosphate almost always remain in solution. Even one of these crystals is an extremely large amount of calcium phosphate compared to what little is required to unbalance the metabolism inside a cell. When fluid is aspirated from an osteoarthritic joint and examined, it shows every kind of calcium phosphate crystal known to medicine. In joints these microscopic crystals abrade and irritate the cartilage in a way that ultimately leads to bony overgrowth, erosions, and loss of tissue. Now, at last, there is some permanent damage to the body.

The fact that the body waits so long before resorting to this means that there is a long-fought, gallant attempt at damage control. Since joints have such a huge capacity to accept these ions, the most essential organs such as the heart, brain, kidneys, and liver, are spared damage from fibromyalgia. When we view the progression of our illness in this manner, we understand that it is fortunate that joints become involved when they do. It is a solution that allows the patient to live, which is nature's priority. And since it takes years for osteoarthritis to become disabling, nature assumes by that time, we will have raised our young to maturity and are thus expendable in the biological order of things.

Although our treatment reverses fibromyalgia and returns our cells to full energy production, it cannot repair damage. The damaged cartilage and the bony spurs of osteoarthritis cannot be changed. This is a compelling reason to begin treatment with guaifenesin as soon as the diagnosis of fibromyalgia is made.

Chapter 11

Pediatric Fibromyalgia

When I was growing up, my nickname was 'Slow as molasses in January.' As I grew older, the sense that I was not like other children deepened; I could not stand still and hold my arms out to have my clothes fitted; I needed more sleep but could not seem to get it; I had little energy and took refuge reading, lying down, on a window seat instead of playing outside. Burying myself in books, I felt the pain and difference of my childhood less acutely, but the guilt was always there; I felt that I was failing everyone around me by not being like them, by not being able to do what they did so effortlessly. My parents, after taking me to the doctor for thyroid tests, concluded that my tiredness was a character trait and not an illness, and I grew up believing them, never having heard anyone say otherwise.

—*Cynthia C., East Lansing, MI*

❧ FACING THE PROBLEM: DOES MY CHILD HAVE FIBROMYALGIA, TOO?

Even when we think we have come to terms with our own fibromyalgia, understand how to treat it, and have started to think about how it has affected our lives, we are terrified to think our children might have it too. Every day I am asked, haltingly, tentatively, by at least one patient: "My daughter has bladder infections and growing pains, do you think she could have fibromyalgia, too?" or "My son used to love sports and now he can't even seem to dress for P.E. Something always seems to be bothering him, do you think he has fibromyalgia?" I am asked about growing pains, headaches, lethargy, and children who go through periods of poor concentration—all in the same anxious tones. None of us want our children to suffer as we have, but deep inside, many of us know our children have the disease too. Before our questions have even been put into words, we know our suspicions are more than suspicions, and I can tell you that most parents are not wrong, they are right on.

With reversal of fibromyalgia we remember our own symptoms. We suddenly recall the pain we had in our side when we were young, headaches we had as teenagers, the irritable bowel syndrome that baffled doctors when we were twelve, growing pains that woke us up in the night, charley horses after gym class or days of fatigue and our inability to concentrate in school—all of these memories come back into our conscious minds during treatment. Through our reversal we are forced to relive parts of our own childhood, and sometimes remember things we had all but forgotten. When we see our own children hurting as we did, we feel guilty for passing our disease onto them. We know what lies ahead for them. We are afraid to tell them what they have because they have seen us suffer so often.

Older children with fibromyalgia already know they are not like other kids. Children cannot articulate their problems or grasp the extent of their deficiencies. How can they understand why it is that today they cannot do their schoolwork but yesterday they could, when grown-ups can barely comprehend it? How can they understand why, when they have slept for a very long time, they are still tired? What does it mean to them when they watch their friends run and play all day and still have energy, when they don't? These are puzzles to the older children, but they learn early to make excuses. It is different for the youngest ones. They have never known another way of life.

We know of one little girl who began painful cycles at the age of two. At night she would wake up crying from the pains in her legs. Her parents soon learned how to interpret her complaints. They would soak her in a warm tub of water, dry her, and massage her legs. This was the only way they could get her back to sleep. That same family has four other children and all of them, like mother and father, have fibromyalgia. It was genetically inescapable that all their children should be affected, and they are. Each of the children had symptoms and findings beginning by the age of four. The only difference is in the extent and severity of their individual symptoms.

Becky, the eldest, was suffering the most by the time we first saw her at the age of eleven. She had intense, daily complaints. She wore a back brace during her waking hours. She visited chiropractors, physiotherapists, and physicians. There were times when she actually had to crawl on the ground to get home from school when her leg pains and weakness got so bad that she could not walk any farther. Becky was so severely involved that I began to suspect she was highly neurotic and using her illness for some gain. I had not yet met any other crawling fibromyalgic or one so young with such severe symptoms. Yet there was more to the story. Becky was also a straight-A student and strikingly intelligent. She learned when she could study most effectively, and rested when she had no choice. She took the pain medications and antidepressants prescribed by her family physician, but even in her sedated state, she continued to excel. Her mother was supportive, and staunchly insisted that Becky was as ill as she seemed to be. Still her mother also kept her in public school, and taught Becky that she had to work through the fatigue and pain as best she could.

Time, Mom, and Becky proved me wrong. Becky responded slowly to guaifenesin because we had to balance her dosage very carefully. Tiny increments in the guaifenesin dosage could set off reversal symptoms with enough intensity to make school attendance impossible. At times, she could not get to class, and had she made it, she would have been unable to sit up for the duration of the period. Becky's personal war continued for over three years; and each tiny victory added to the rest became a battle won. Today this remarkable young woman is in her senior year in college and remains a straight-A student. She has only minor cycles of fibromyalgia reversal. Becky says that she will never forget how she once crawled to get home from school. This marvelous young woman plans to turn her remarkable story and mental gifts to health sciences and the healing of others. The medical profession should be proud to have her.

When my younger son, Sean, was small, his father took him to a pediatric rheumatologist who diagnosed him with a "pain syndrome." The doctor hesitated to make the diagnosis of fibromyalgia, he said, because Sean did not seem to have a sleep disorder. This doctor, who admitted he had never heard of guaifenesin, was willing to write a prescription on the spot for Elavil and Flexeril—for a seven-year-old child who was far from being in intractable pain. I could not believe this. He did not even know what was wrong with my son except that he was in pain, and admitted it, yet he was willing to change the chemistry of a seven-year-old child's brain.

—C.C., Los Angeles

As heartwarming as Becky's story is, there are many sad ones. I have known too many children who have ended up as invalids because of their fibromyalgia. Some parents, frightened by the plight of their children, become overprotective. Their children are kept home at the slightest provocation, become inactive, and soon no longer have friends or participate in activities. The entire family begins to revolve around the symptoms of the child, who is soon given narcotics for pain and hypnotics for sleep. The child lives in an altered state, barely able to function. When pain medications are no longer effective, their desperate parents call doctors at all hours requesting even stronger medications. These parents have acquiesced to a life of drug habituation for their children.

Many absences from school eventually make these children unable to compete academically. The student falls further behind, and may never catch up. Occasionally parents manage to wrench home-schooling tutors out of their local school districts. Although this helps the children academically, their inability to take on extracurricular activities deprives them of crucial social interaction and development during their teenage years. They become defined by the list of things they cannot do.

Time is oddly suspended in the present for these families. There is never a discussion about the future when mother and father will be too old to continue as caretakers. Adulthood does not end the drug dependence or the isolation. Parents suddenly have a young adult on their hands who can no longer be carried on the family medical insurance and is both unemployable and ineligible for disability benefits because he or she has never worked.

Recounting these stories brings to mind a little boy I remember vividly named Joe. When we met, he was sick, and afraid of doctors and of more pain. As time progressed, I learned to appreciate his good qualities. We became friends. At one appointment he brought a poem of gratitude he had written especially for me. I hung it on my office wall.

Joe and his family moved away. When he came back to see me a few years later, he was changed. His mother and her new doctors had started him on narcotic pain medications. These were the very drugs I had refused to prescribe for him because of their addictive potential. Narcotics had quickly become his new friends and provided instant relief, as opposed to the slow improvement I had offered with guaifenesin. Joe had missed too much school and needed a doctor's note so that he would not be held back. I don't know what happened to him after that because his mother chose to continue with doctors who would prescribe the drugs that I would not. I don't think Joe ever became the basketball player he dreamed of becoming.

Recalling Joe saddens me. Becky's story, on the other hand, will always make me smile, and it partially offsets the other. She owes a great deal to her mother, who did not shy away from treatment with a denial of her daughter's illness, or make it an option for her to quit when things were not easy. Both these stories underscore the point of this chapter. *We must make the diagnosis of fibromyalgia in the young as soon as possible, and treat their illness.*

It is a simple fact: children have not had the disease as long as adults have. There is less disease to reverse so it will take less time for them to recover. We must pay attention to their complaints and the few signs they can offer. As parents with the disease, we have the bonus of being able to recognize ourselves at that age to help us with our children. We can change our guilt to satisfaction knowing that we have spared our children from what we have been through. Despite our genetic transfer, our children can lead normal, full, and productive lives. As parents we must take charge and demand a diagnosis and effective treatment. We must do whatever it takes and not give up. Our children are watching us and will learn from our example.

I do not remember a time when I did not have headaches. Since my mother had always suffered from migraines, my headaches seemed to be part of my destiny. The pain in my head was, at least, taken to be real by my family. Not so by the outside world, in which, during my adolescence, I would often hear: just relax, lie down in a dark room for a few minutes, take an aspirin. Fasting glucose tests, an electroencephalogram, an electrocardiogram, and other tests at the university clinic showed nothing. I had migraines, and not much could be done beyond living with them. Expensive shiatsu and acupuncture gave me sporadic relief but no more than that. I lived my life around my pain, as frustrated as my doctors. I hid my pain as best I could, but I could not hide it from those closest to me. By the time my daughter was three, every week I was taking a bottle of naproxen sodium and Tylenol, and as much sumatriptan as I could get my doctors and medical plan to pro-

vide, and yet I was still helplessly spending my afternoons on the couch. I had severe headaches every day, and most of them were migraines. I felt isolated by my pain, unable to even begin to communicate to anyone what my life was like, and increasingly devastated and guilty from the effect my pain was having on my family.
— *Cynthia C., East Lansing, MI*

❀ FIBROMYALGIA IN CHILDREN

I remember clearly the moment I knew my son had fibromyalgia. And it was not his complaints of pains or nervousness that tipped me off. I didn't know that children do not normally complain of headaches, because I had them all my life. I didn't know there was no such thing as growing pains. His aches and pains did not disrupt his life, and I did not think much about them either. But one day I was standing in the doorway watching his trumpet lesson, and I heard his trumpet teacher say: "At this point I shouldn't have to tell you how to play a B note." And I looked at my son's face, and I knew that at that moment he had no more idea how to play a B on a trumpet than I did, although he did know. All the times in my childhood when I was yelled at, told I knew things I could not bring out of my mind because my mind just wouldn't always work to produce them on demand, came flooding back. I knew then and there Malcolm had fibromyalgia too, and I would have to get him help.
— *Claudia Craig Marek*

If you or anyone in your family has fibromyalgia, look as objectively as possible at your child. No doctor on earth will ever know that little person as well as you do. But what should you look for? Pain is one complaint to listen for. Kids just don't make up pain very often, and when they do it's something transparent like a tummy ache to get out of something they don't want to do. Children are relatively inarticulate and will not usually say more than "it hurts" or "I have a headache." As we have said, the youngest ones will not even recall a time when they did not have some of their symptoms. To them they are normal, so they will try to tell you only about the bigger or newer pains.

Are your children tired in the mornings beyond what seems normal and when they have had plenty of sleep? Do they take spontaneous naps at times when other children are out playing? Can you tell when they are having difficulty with memory or concentration? Can they do their homework with ease one night, but find it impossible the next? Do they have abdominal pain, constipation, and diarrhea? Does your daughter have bladder infections, painful urination, or pelvic pain? Are there growing pains centered in and about the knees? We have even wondered about colic in babies, but there are no follow-up studies describing these children or demographic studies of the prevalence of fibromyalgia in their parents.

Older children have gradually realized they are different. They know they do not have the same stamina as their friends. They are aware of brain-haze days when their schoolbooks might as well have been written in a foreign language. They have times when their backpack suddenly seems too heavy and is painful to carry. They are dizzy and exhausted for no particular reason, and their eyes do not always focus. For some it is that glassy look that teachers see and attribute to deliberate inattention. Assuming that these symptoms are due to growing or to being a normal, lazy teenager may be a disservice, especially if at other times your child seems perfectly fine.

Children with FMS often cycle from an early age, even from preschool years, with achy days that put them into their whiny and irritable moods. They later test their parents with complaints of aching around their legs and knees. These are commonly labeled growing pains, especially by grandparents. These leg pains seem to occur most often around the ages of eight to ten, but sometimes start as early as five years old. They come and go without rhyme or reason and may continue over a span of a few months and rarely for as long as a year or two. A few adults insist they remember that their attacks cycled over as much as a five-year span.

We were surprised when we were sent a paper written in 1928 by a family practitioner. He described children with growing pains, "great mental and body fatigue," cold extremities, and "feeble digestion," along with several other symptoms that make us think of fibromyalgia. He treated his patients with great success using a tree bark extract called guaiacum. Several years later this guaiacum was purified into guaiacolate and even later became an ingredient in some cough preparations. Over twenty years ago this same medicine became our guaifenesin![25]

We find when we quiz our adult patients at the time of their first visit that a history of growing pains is exremely common. Since these are often the earliest recognizable symptoms of fibromyalgia, they help us to determine the onset of the disease. Yet calling these pains, "growing pains" is actually a misnomer, because the pains begin before the great growth spurt of approaching puberty. During the growth spurt itself, the body requires huge amounts of everything, including phosphates.

Since the body uses all available phosphate during this period, it is often almost symptom-free, and no new areas are affected.

When growth slows down again in the later teenage years, complaints relating to fibromyalgia begin again. Since most patients are female, premenstrual symptoms predominate. Headaches may make their first appearance at this time, as fibromyalgics begin their adolescent cycling. Women frequently tell us it was about this time that they first became aware of their physical deficiencies. They were unable to keep up with their friends in physical activities. In the gym or on the athletic field, although they might have displayed ability, they soon tired and began to lag behind. They began to be conscious of a lack of stamina. The thought of performing physical activities eventually terrorized them because of a marked increase in muscular pains that night or the next day. Many women say that it was at this age that they stopped participating in any physical activity except mandatory physical education classes.

Over the years, we have treated many children under the age of sixteen. My three daughters suffered their first cycles at the ages of eleven, thirteen, and sixteen respectively. My coauthor Claudia's sons were both diagnosed before seven, the age when we began their treatment. Her younger son Sean, a gifted athlete, had a high pain threshold and complained of only minor aches, but we soon realized that his bouts of diarrhea were manifestations of fibromyalgia. These were the first symptoms of the irritable bowel syndrome. When I examined him, I found the widespread body lumps and bumps that clinched the diagnosis of fibromyalgia. We were all rewarded when his irritable bowel quickly cleared with treatment. The elder of the two, Malcolm, my guaifenesin guinea pig, was fully articulate (seemingly from birth) and was able to express himself very forcefully. He had the usual mass of symptoms, including those that affect the brain, musculoskeletal system, and gastrointestinal tract. We have since begun treating a family that includes two young girls who, like their mother, have vulvar pain as their prime complaint.

From the large number we have treated, we have learned that although their problems are the same, children present with as many different complaints as adult patients do. Fibromyalgia affects the same systems in children as in adults, but children pay much less attention to the overall picture, and the history and continuum is frequently wanting. As parents we must find doctors who are willing to listen to us about our children and be willing to do something to help. Pediatricians should also learn to conduct a body search and begin mapping the swollen fibromyalgic lesions. The affected areas of fibromyalgia are easily discovered with this technique, which greatly facilitates making the diagnosis. This is especially valuable in the younger patients who are often unable to describe their symptoms.

❧ TREATMENT

I think I had FMS for about 20 years. . . . Looking back into my childhood, I can now see the very first symptoms beginning around age nine or ten. . . . My daughter Jill is sixteen years old. Since my diagnosis, I realized that she had some of the symptoms of FMS. The symptoms became more and more pronounced and I finally realized about two years ago that she also had it. At that point I was unwilling to tell her this. How could I tell a fourteen-year-old adolescent that she was going to be in as much pain as her mother . . . without any knowledge of a cure? At that point in my illness, I was in excruciating pain, cried every day and didn't know what to do for myself.

I started guaifenesin under Dr. St. Amand's guidance in October 1996. He was incredibly gentle, helpful, sincere, but most of all he gave me *hope*. Once I realized that guaifenesin worked, I finally had the courage to tell my daughter what I suspected . . . that she also had FMS. I confirmed her diagnosis with a doctor and we agreed that she would start the guaifenesin once school was over in June.

No matter how much pain I am in, it does not compare to the emotional pain of seeing my daughter in pain with FMS. Even worse is that I know what her pain feels like . . . because I have it too. I now realize that Jill has probably had FMS for about 5 or 6 years . . . we just didn't know it at the time.

—*Aileen Goldberg, New York City*

There is no need to go into great detail about the treatment of children with guaifenesin, since it is the same as for adults. We often start them at 300 mg twice a day and gradually raise the dose until reverse cycling begins. Guaifenesin is available in 300 mg capsules with the trade name Pediatric Sprinkles. The net cost is higher than comparable doses would be using the adult preparations. Though it is a more expensive way to buy the drug, parents rarely make this an issue. If a child is unable to swallow half tablets of the 600 mg size, they may be able to handle the slicker capsule. If not, the capsules can be opened and poured into a drink or spread on food. As with adults, the doses should be spaced roughly twelve hours apart.

It is sometimes wiser to delay the initiation of treatment until the start of school vacation or the long winter break. This is usually easier on parents because they can give the child more time to rest and avoid facing the simultaneous struggle with the first reversal cycles, school, and homework. If the drug is started at the beginning of a vacation, most children will have experienced noticeable improvement by the time classes resume. There is obviously no reason to delay treatment in a preschooler. It may be best to cancel music or dance lessons for a month or two at the beginning of treatment. This naturally depends on the severity of the child's illness and his individual stamina. If a break from some activities seems necessary, assure your child that he is getting well and will soon resume his normal routine. You can add activities back one by one without waiting for your youngster to get totally well. Children can cope quite well even when they are only partially better. It will also help them to remain active and not miss out on too many things.

It is difficult to watch children suffer, especially for the parent who has transmitted the defective gene. The first few reversal cycles will be painful, yes, but if a child is not in school, he can be helped with bed rest, warm baths, and Tylenol or Advil as needed. Benadryl is available in pediatric strengths and can help a child in pain fall asleep. Children should be encouraged to stay active, play with their friends, and understand that there is nothing wrong with them that time won't fix. The parent walks a bit of a tightrope at this point, providing compassion and yet remaining firm in the resolve that some symptoms must be endured. It will sometimes seem that you need the wisdom of Solomon and the patience of Job to accomplish this and still hold your child to certain standards of achievement and behavior, but in truth common sense and listening to your child are an admirable substitute for the above. Older children quickly learn to work when they are feeling better and rest when they are tired or in pain. Smaller children will not understand what is happening to them during bouts of fibromyalgia, but you will have plenty of chances to explain the illness as they get older.

Most children test the system when they are feeling well. At one point or another, expect them to stop taking their medication. All of our children have done it, even Malcolm, the original guinea-kid, despite his pride at being the first person we treated with guaifenesin. He must have felt that great surge of invincibility that can only come with being a teenager. Rest assured, they will find their way back to that bottle of guaifenesin on the medicine shelf when symptoms start again. Luckily, since they are young and have not fallen far behind, they respond quickly, and it will not take long to make up for lost ground.

Guaifenesin is safe at any age. The road back from fibromyalgia is more easily traveled in the early stages. We must learn to diagnose the illness sooner than has been our habit, for the sake of our children. We are fortunate to have a medicine that can quickly restore them to normal. Those of us with fibromyalgia will inevitably reflect on our own lives. We will wonder how we would have been different if we had had the opportunity for an early diagnosis and treatment. For most of us, life would certainly have included more happiness and far less wasted years of suffering. Yet as parents we also know that if the memory of our suffering gives us the strength to help our children, it was not entirely wasted.

PART III

❦

STRATEGIES FOR THE ROAD BACK

Unlike the chapters included in Part II, the following chapters are not specifically about treating fibromyalgia or its syndromes. Rather, they are about practical, everyday matters—coping with your job, your family, your home, and your other medications and treatments.

We hope that the information and suggestions in the following chapters will help you cope with the disease on a daily basis. Undoubtedly, you will learn some things that your doctor has not told you, or that you have not learned through other sources. We hope you will benefit from the information and that it will help you while you're waiting to begin (or are in the early stages of) your guaifenesin treatment.

Chapter 12

Medical Band-Aids: Currently Accepted
Treatments for Fibromyalgia—What
You Don't Know *Can* Hurt You

> Neither my general practitioner nor my rheumatologist would
> talk to me about guaifenesin (to treat my fibromyalgia). My
> rheumatologist told me I would have to learn to live with the pain
> and illness for the rest of my life. I agree that this may happen, but
> if there is anything that can help slow it down or reverse it, why
> not try? No medication can be any worse than some of the med-
> ications I have tried.
>
> —*Bonnie Jean, Phoenix, AZ*

There is no mystery to the standard method of treating fibromyalgia. The party line is echoed throughout medical literature, and little or no dissent is heard. Papers describing
protocols different from the accepted party line are often refused publication for several reasons. Medical journals usually
require double-blind studies with normal controls. This is
quite impossible for the practicing physician to accomplish.
He cannot give a placebo, or sugar pill, to half of the patients
who come to him and pay for treatment, nor can he perform
tests on people who are not ill. The peer review process is an-

other obstacle. Before a medical/professional article is approved for publication, the manuscript is sent to experts in the field for comments and approval. These "peers," often editors of journals, are wary of new approaches. They are especially leery of ideas that arise from those not in academia, where research is expected to originate. What they say goes, and few question the system. On the whole, it is a proper procedure that has been designed for patient safety.

At times however, the system seems unresponsive. It is unfortunate when effective treatments are lost for lack of publication because they are only based on a lifetime of medical observation and cannot fit into the proper slot. What is learned from working with thousands of patients should carry some weight. Conclusions reached during an extended period of observation may prove correct in the long run and they may anticipate by many years what the system will later confirm as fact. There are no journals dedicated to observations made by practicing physicians. Vast hands-on experience should have a value, but often no forum is provided and the findings die with the observer. We have written this book because we have no other way to help. We can only reach patients who will, in turn, reach physicians, quite the reverse of the usual order for the treatment of illness!

🐚 THE ACCEPTED TREATMENT

It may well be better not to treat patients with our well-known but hardly effective armamentarium of drugs. . . . Treatments with antidepressants, tricyclics, formal exercise programs—particularly because they

do not seem to work—prolong medicalization and dependency, the opposite of what we should wish to
accomplish.

—*Frederick Wolfe, M.D.,*
Journal of Rheumatology [26]

So what is the accepted treatment for fibromyalgia? We already
know that it is largely ineffective since disability claims, alternative treatments, and self-help groups abound. It is also true
that for many people, the deplorable choices they have been
offered by doctors are no improvement over simply suffering
from the disease in silence.

The established and accepted plan for treating fibromyalgia is:

• Relieve the patient's pain as much as possible.

• Maintain a positive attitude about the patient's chance for
recovery.

• Help the patient get some sleep.

• Tell patients to exercise because it will make them feel
better.

• Help patients who cannot work obtain disability.

On the surface, I cannot imagine anyone quarreling with
any of these goals. They are lofty and simple enough and, were
they possible, would be the answer to a patient's misery. Or
would they? Looking more deeply, one cannot escape noticing
that despite their appeal to common sense, not one of them
aims at altering the metabolic malfunction that is the basis of

fibromyalgia. None of them will keep a patient from getting worse, and none will help a patient get back to normal. Let's look more closely to better understand what these guidelines mean to a fibromyalgic.

Pain

By the time patients visit doctors they have more pain than they can handle by themselves. The brain gives pain priority over other sensations and feelings because it is a warning sign that damage is occurring. It's designed to demand immediate action with the goal of preventing further injury. Thus, relieving pain is certainly a noble goal. Patients will have tried the over-the-counter analgesics—aspirin and acetaminophen—and usually the nonsteroidal, anti-inflammatory drugs as well (ibuprofen, naproxen, and others). They may have already begun prescription medications: a muscle relaxant such as carisoprodol (Soma) or cyclobenzaprine (Flexeril), or a stronger pain tablet such as propoxyphene (Darvon). The initial relief most patients experience with these medications wears off rather quickly. More than a few will have raised their dosages steadily higher. Medical literature tells both patient and physician this is appropriate. Eventually, however, the sympathetic doctor doesn't know what else to suggest.

Now the soggy-eyed, droopy-lidded, slouched-over, and largely unrelieved patient moves on to a new doctor's examination table. After a brief introduction, the patient begins a litany of the various routes taken by satanic pain, and how miserable he is as a result. Simply taking a history alone will fill the next twenty to thirty minutes. In a testimonial to the age of computers and copying machines, many patients helpfully bring ten-page documents detailing every doctor they have seen, every medication that did nothing much, and on what date each of their many symptoms appeared. There are surgery reports and gruesome details of accidents. Sheets of laboratory results—tests done on every obtainable bodily fluid—are next, sometimes with a hair or saliva analysis thrown in for good measure. Most of these tests are normal, but here and there a slight deviation may be circled. Some patients bring the results of X rays, MRIs, ultrasounds, and scans, and a pile of reports describing the findings of a variety of medical examiners. They look at the new doctor expectantly. They have done their part in good faith. It's the doctor's turn now.

What do you suppose the I've-heard-it-all-before doctor is thinking? He knows the patients in his waiting room are rechecking their watches and by now have even finished last year's newsmagazines. Soon they will be plaintively asking his receptionist: "Is the doctor almost ready for me?" There is probably a patient in the adjoining exam room freezing to death in a piece of crumpled paper euphemistically referred to as a "gown."

The frustrated physician must think quickly. "She needs pain relief; she's already tried a bunch of over-the-counter drugs. OK, I know what I've got to do." Out comes the pad, and the least powerful of the pain drugs is prescribed. Propoxyphene (Darvocet-N), tramadol (Ultram), isometheptene mucate (Midrin), or perhaps a more potent nonsteroidal anti-inflammatory such as diclofenac (Cataflam) or etodolac (Lodine)—whatever is not on the patient's already-done-that-and-it-doesn't-work list. If the patient has never used these drugs before, they will give some modicum of relief before they too are relegated to the growing list of what doesn't work.

It won't be long before the physician has to pull out his prescription pad once more. It's time to step up the attack with the bigger guns. The opiate derivatives will certainly do the job better. Now come the codeine combinations—Tylenol No. 3, Vicodin, Lorcet, or any of the various brands of hydrocodones. If patients can tolerate their side effects, the pain is at least dulled, as these drugs usually provide a lot of relief at first. Hydrocodone will eventually give way to the more potent time-released oxycontin; then to patches or drips of increasingly stronger compounds. More doctors are finding the use of methadone acceptable though they admit "nearly all patients on opioids become physically dependent."[27]

Unless the fundamental cause of FMS itself is treated, the pain will eventually break through all analgesics, at least partially. When relief is no longer significant, narcotics can be used in greater strengths. But here comes the catch. The real danger is that the patient has begun a vicious cycle of feeling pain, achieving temporary relief, and developing tolerance to very potent medications.

Physicians do remember, for the most part, to warn their patients that narcotics are habituating, but too often, they fail to give a clear description of what that actually means and what a narcotic is. They continue to write prescriptions for a hundred tablets and a few refills. This facilitates escalating consumption, because at the point where the same dosage no longer affords relief and a demanding brain screams for "a bit more, just this time," a patient has enough on hand to do this.

After patients have taken these drugs for a few months, it's very difficult to stop using them, even on days when they feel better. Any attempt to decrease consumption will result in increased pain sensations. This is called dependence and occurs because the body has adapted to the medicine and wants to continue to get it. To this end, it will reproduce the physical symptoms for which it was given the drug. Patients will perceive that the pain level produced by their disease still requires the same dose of medication, and will continue taking it.

In medicine we sometimes play with words. "Habituation" and "dependence" versus "addiction" is an example of this. Physicians like to have clear separations—black and white suits us much better than gray. Physicians (and patients) are most comfortable when facts and entities fall into distinct, definable categories. When they appear as a smooth, continuous spectrum and imperceptibly blend from one level to another, we are most uncomfortable. We know that we are supposed to ease pain; it is part of our oath. But *primum no nocere*—above all do no harm, should supersede our need to be heroes and curb all pain no matter what. Physicians should understand the escalating drug dependency into which we are sending our patients. Instead of prescribing temporary analgesia, we should think about our credo: *For chronic diseases, do not give addictive drugs.* We should make it our primary business to treat disease and not symptoms.

Many of you fibromyalgics will want to put this book down in anger just about now, but don't. Hear my message. Treat the cause of your disease instead of just the mental and physical pains. You have been searching for good health— here is a chance. You can help yourself and avoid getting caught somewhere in the gray zone between habituation and addiction.

An Overview of Medications Commonly Used for Fibromyalgia

> I am the original poster boy for what can go wrong
> when on certain antidepressants. They, the old docs,
> started me out on 10 mg, and by the time it was over
> I was at 200 mg a day. It took weeks of pain, grief, and
> very scary thoughts before it flushed out of my system.
> We are not depressed by FMS; we are depressed be-
> cause we have never been treated properly and fairly
> until now.
>
> —*Joel S., Wisconsin*

There are no pain medications in the *Physicians' Desk Ref-erence* that are indicated as safe for long-term use, for chronic pain, or for pain that lasts longer than six months. This is largely because the medications themselves are not considered "safe" for everyday use because of the potential side effects. But for other, very real, physical reasons, chronic pain is much more difficult to treat than acute pain.

Acute pain from trauma floods the body with hormones and releases endorphins, the body's own natural painkillers. Endorphins, which are naturally occurring opioids, occupy the body's pain receptors and are why we do not feel acute pain at the time of an injury.

The body is not geared to remain in this energy-intensive emergency mode for long. When the pain messages continue for a long period, the body becomes desensitized to them. After a while, less endorphins are produced to counter the same level of pain—this is one of the reasons why fibromyal-gics are thought by some doctors to be oversensitive to all pain.

"The estimated risk of developing end-stage renal disease

in habitual users of analgesic agents, who are described as using analgesics daily for five years or longer, is the same as that for smokers to develop carcinoma of the lung, namely, 2 in 1000."[28]

So if a patient eschews narcotics for chronic pain, what is left? Acetaminophen is one option, but studies are accumulating showing that acetaminophen (Tylenol) can lead to renal or hepatic damage if taken regularly over several years. Nonsteroidal anti-inflammatory drugs (NSAIDs) are another choice, as they are commonly used for their analgesic effect in addition to their use as an anti-inflammatory. Keep in mind though, that with FMS there is no inflammation present. NSAIDs are no safer than acetaminophen for long-term use. They are known to cause stomach bleeding and can cause liver damage both in the short and long term. Newer studies of both NSAIDs and acetaminophen suggest that they may interfere with basic energy production. This and the fact that NSAIDs disrupt the deepest stage of sleep in some patients are special concerns for fibromyalgics.

Other types of drugs and antidepressants are also used for making fibromyalgics more comfortable. Since the mid-1980s they have been used in low doses—lower than can be used to control depression—for fibromyalgia. Yet, as Doctor Don L. Goldenberg, M.D., one of the nation's leading specialists, points out in "A Review of the Role of Tricyclic Medications in the Treatment of Fibromyalgia Syndrome," "only 25 to 35 percent of patients have a meaningful response to these medications."[29] The fact that doctors have latched on to these drugs and prescribe them so abundantly despite these unpromising statistics shows how desperate they are to find something that may help. In the patients for whom these drugs are effective, sleep patterns may be helped or restored, depression eased, and pain perception decreased up to fifty percent. The original tricyclic medications and the newer specific serotonin reuptake inhibitors and serotonin and norephinepherine reuptake inhibitors are all prescribed. In general their effects are similar, except no pain reduction has been shown with Serzone, one of the serotonin reuptake inhibitors.

While the above paragraph sounds promising, there is actually more to the story. Antidepressants have no lasting benefits for fibromyalgia, even though some pain is masked and depression may lessen, at least initially. Their effectiveness seems to lessen after about nine weeks of use, and in any case, the disease marches on and symptoms will burst through the drug suppression at some point. Doses should not be titrated upwards. Studies have shown that if these drugs do not work at a reasonably low dose, they will not do much more at a higher dose. Antidepressants such as Prozac may also disrupt Stage 4 sleep in some patients, leaving them feeling "wired."

> Although tricyclic medications, notably low doses of amitriptyline and cyclobenzaprine, have been beneficial in controlled therapeutic trials in fibromyalgia, overall effectiveness in patients has not been impressive. Patient self-rating of medicinal therapy has been no better than such nonmedicinal treatments as physical and chiropractic therapy. Only 30–40 percent of our patients described medications as very effective. In the only long-term longitudinal study reported in FMS we surveyed 39 patients for three consecutive years. Although 83 percent of them continued to take

some medications, usually multiple, during the three
years, only 20 percent felt well.

—Don L. Goldenberg, M.D.,
Journal of Rheumatology[30]

Muscle relaxants and antianxiety drugs round out the list
of the most common prescription drugs used by fibromyalgics.
Double-blind studies have been hard to conduct because the
side effects of these drugs are so obvious. Most patients can tolerate them in only very limited quantities because of the level
of fatigue they induce. As with the other medications we have
mentioned, for patients who can tolerate them, they provide a
certain amount of relief from muscle spasm and may help with
sleep. Morning drowsiness and mental fogginess are the two
main reasons why patients discontinue them.

The fact that patients take vast amounts of drugs and supplements and in so many combinations is ample proof that
none of these substances are very effective. When patients ask
about this drug or that, my stock answer is that I have no opinion because what seems to help one patient may have no effect
for another. I tell them that if there were one good answer for
controlling pain and fatigue, everyone would know it, and
that's what everyone would be taking. It is important for both
patients and doctors to know that there is no single prescription drug that is capable of taking away all the pain. Instead, I
urge patients to take guaifenesin and use their limited energy
to get well, instead of searching for a chemical Band-Aid to
mask their symptoms. In general, it seems to me and most of
my patients that when the amount of relief afforded is weighed
against potential side effects, most of these solutions are unap-
pealing.

In response to the lobbying efforts of the multi-billion-dollar "dietary supplement" industry, Congress in 1994 exempted their products from FDA regulation. . . . Since then these products have flooded the market, subject only to the scruples of their manufacturers. They may contain the substances listed on the label in the amounts claimed, but they need not, and there is no one to prevent their sale if they don't. In an analysis of ginseng products, for example, the amount of active ingredient in each pill varied by as much as a factor of 10 among brands that were labeled as containing the same amount. Some brands contained none at all. . . . The only legal requirement in the sale of such products is that they not be promoted as preventing or treating disease. To comply with that stipulation, their labeling has risen to an art-form of doublespeak.

—*Marcia Angell, M.D., Jerome P. Kassirer, M.D.,*
New England Journal of Medicine[31]

It is not within the scope of this book to write about herbal medications and whether or not they are safe or effective. Since plant products will block guaifenesin, they are a moot point to us. In other places in this book we have questioned the wisdom of taking many compounds to receive a potential benefit from one or two. We have also pointed out that the FDA does not regulate the quality of herbal medications and the veracity of their claims. Several recent articles in medical journals and newsmagazines have disclosed that many of these medications are contaminated and can vary tremendously in concentration. Since patients who wish to take them will not be seeking information in this book, there seems no need to delve further into the matter here.

Hormones such as DHEA, thyroid, and estrogen, which will not block guaifenesin, are also used by some doctors in the treatment of fibromyalgia. As an endocrinologist, I strongly suggest patients do extensive research before even considering any of these. Hormones have many effects on the body, and at this point, not all of them are known or completely understood. Even less is known about what the effect will be of raising levels above a patient's own normal hormone level. Thyroid hormone in excess of normal levels is known to cause the loss of bone density, and the relationship between hormones such as estrogen and some cancers is still being debated. Patients should also steer clear of animal-origin supplements as well as raw gland extracts such as that of the thymus gland. Tests have shown that thymus gland extract can transfer infectious parasites from one species to another through a mechanism called prion transfer.

Vitamins and supplements in anything other than great moderation should also send up warning flags. Very little is known about consuming large quantities of any vitamins, and there is evidence that some of them, particularly the fat-soluble ones, could be dangerous. As far as we know, minerals will not block guaifenesin because they are not of plant origin, but they can interfere with some prescription medications. Calcium is known to block the action of some antibiotics, and magnesium can block the prescription drug Neurontin.

I should tell you that not only have I improved due to guaifenesin, I have also thrown off all the other stuff I was on. Now, I use no sleeping pills, no antidepressants, no steroids, and I used to think I needed all three of them for the rest of my life. I only take a little Tylenol now and then for headaches, and of course, guaifenesin.

—*Jeri Lynn, California*

We treat our patients with only one simple medication—guaifenesin. It has been around in some form for years (first mention: guaicum, 1530 A.D.) and is devoid of side effects. We are especially pleased when new patients come to us taking no medications. When they take no other drugs, minerals, vitamins or other supplements, there can be no confusion. When they get well, they know why. They will never find themselves in the sad world of polypharmacy.

Sleep

Difficulty falling asleep and staying asleep long enough to reach the Stage 4 phase of restorative sleep is the first major hurdle that we face in dealing with the other symptoms of FMS. I absolutely cannot nap no matter how hard I try, and going to sleep at night requires a ritual of sleep aids, a calming atmosphere, total darkness in the room, numerous pillows piled around my body, a light-weight cover. I would like to trade a day with a normal person who goes out like a light, sleeps deeply and wakes refreshed. Oh I wish. . . .

—*Elizabeth R., Georgia*

The desire for restful sleep eventually leads exhausted fibromyalgics to demand sleeping pills from physicians. A new mattress, expensive pillows, and white noise tapes have not made a difference. Pre-bedtime rituals such as warm baths, dimmed lights, soothing music, or meditation that may have helped initially are no longer working. I know from my own experience that nighttime inactivity stiffened my already-contracted muscles, tendons, and ligaments. Every time I lay in one position for a few minutes, my pain would mount progressively, at first subliminally, just enough to make me restless. Eventually, the pain intensity increased and awakened me from whatever sleep stage I had managed to reach. My nights were a bit like the Indianapolis 500, moving to and fro, navigating for position. I could make my victory lap only if I got a good night's rest. As I recall, I rarely won.

I urge my patients to consider an over-the-counter sleeping aid—diphenhydramine (an antihistamine known by the brand name Benadryl). It makes one drowsy and is not habit-forming. It is safe, even for children, and is often allowed by obstetricians during pregnancy. Diphenhydramine is most commonly marketed as a 25 mg capsule, and the dosage can be titrated up to 300 mg a night. This medication is the sleep-inducing ingredient in over-the-counter compounds such as Tylenol PM, Sominex, and Unisom. It is documented to help patients reach delta, or deep-sleep, levels. In some patients, antihistamines cause jitters and excitability; obviously, they should not attempt to use this compound for sleep.

Melatonin is a hormone released by the pineal gland. It has many effects in the body, where it eventually becomes serotonin. As of this writing it seems safe and helps many people to sleep. Melatonin functions by resetting the body clock, and studies have shown it to be quite effective in controlling jet lag. Levels of this hormone decline with age, which may be one of the reasons why elderly people may have trouble sleeping. Its safety has not been established for children or teenagers because they produce large amounts naturally. It is my observation that it seems to work best in older patients.

The sublingual form of melatonin provides quicker action and allows for smaller dosages. It acts faster because it's placed under the tongue, where it dissolves quickly and goes directly into the bloodstream instead of through the digestive tract. We have found added benefits by using combinations of this hormone with diphenhydramine. There is some new evidence that melatonin may also make amitriptyline (Elavil) more effective. Physicians and patients should understand that if a patient has been taking prescription sleeping pills, melatonin will not work immediately. Patients should be encouraged to wean off their sleeping pill by gradually lowering the dose and at the same time beginning melatonin. In some patients melatonin causes depression, and if it does, it is best to discontinue use.

If patients cannot tolerate the above compounds, we turn to prescription medications in desperation. The next step is to give patients sedatives, or sleeping pills. These vary greatly in their habit-forming propensities, yet all have the potential to create dependence. If my patients insist on using them, I suggest taking the tiniest amounts possible and avoiding nightly use. Although this results in less sleep on alternate nights, it is much better in the long run.

Side effects are also a problem with sedatives. They depress the central nervous system, causing a morning hangover. Fibromyalgics have difficulty functioning in the morning, and this may be a serious problem. Sleeping pills also cause a rebound effect the next day, usually in the late afternoon. If patients yield to this drowsiness and take a nap, sleep is much more difficult a few hours later at bedtime, creating a vicious cycle.

It is extremely important for patients to realize that many medications, including sedatives, muscle relaxants, tranquilizers, antianxiety drugs, antidepressants, and narcotic pain medications, add significantly to an already-overwhelming fatigue. It's a toss-up whether or not the added sleep they provide can produce enough energy to overcome their sapping effects. The list of medications that can cause somnolence is long, and many patients are taking more than one of them. I urge all patients with unrelenting fatigue to review their medications with a pharmacist and check for this common contributing factor. Over-the-counter nonsteroidal anti-inflammatories and analgesics may also contribute to decreased energy production, according to the newest studies.

Although we've learned that it is better to take only guaifenesin, for many it is difficult to do so. Many of us started on a number of different medications. I was diagnosed with FMS in 1988 and have been on plenty of medications since then. My symptoms began in 1977. I was taking Elavil for three years and Ambien for two. I tried to stop taking both of these a number of times before guaifenesin but I was in such sad shape I would have to start up again. I very slowly weaned myself off the Elavil. That was not very hard to do. I had no real reaction from stopping. I was concerned with the Ambien because I needed to sleep, so I cut way back, usually only taking 1/4 of a tablet at night except when I was feeling well. Then I stopped taking it. The first few nights I used Benadryl, it made me very groggy. Then I tried melatonin and got the same results. I also tried a combination that made me groggy too. So, after a week of messing around I went to bed without anything and I fell asleep just fine. . . .

—*Linda P., Ohio*

Common Medications with Fatigue or Somnolence as a Side Effect

Antihistamines (Atarax and Benadryl); sleeping pills (Ambien, ProSom, etc.); antidepressants (Elavil and others); muscle relaxants (Flexeril, Soma); allergy pills, including Hismanal; blood pressure medications (Inderal, Cardura) and antispasmotics; anticholinergics (Librax); pain medications (Ultram, codeine, Darvocet, etc.); antianxiety drugs (Valium, Centrax, etc.) and tranquilizers (Sinequan, Klonopin). Most of these medications also list depression and weakness as side effects. In addition, tranquilizers can also shorten the attention span, decrease ability to concentrate, and give a muted sense of reality.

Exercise

> I also have a problem with pain the day after [sexual] intercourse which, just like any other type of exercise, makes me hurt for days and may send me into a flare.
>
> —*B.J., Arizona*

Exercise is an especially lauded part of the established treatment plan for fibromyalgia. It is near and dear to the heart of many researchers and practitioners. Most urge stretching and pool workouts. I heartily endorse these types of gentle exercise that do not overstress the patient's body.

There are also physicians who urge patients to do more strenuous aerobic exercise, despite the fact that most patients cannot tolerate them without paying a heavy price later. It is our contention that the aches and pains of fibromyalgia are caused by intracellular metabolic debris that accumulates due to an inherited genetic defect. As long as this debris remains in the cells, they stay in the alert state, in perpetual calcium overdrive, in effect participating in a low-grade workout without reprieve. This occurs in all cells of the body, not just in muscles. The brain, endocrine organs, skin, and intestine can also be thought of as overexercised units. Heavy exercise, which adds markedly to this debris, only exacerbates the condition and makes impossible demands. Malfunction ensues in the form of more pain, fatigue, and metabolic ineptness in other tissues.

The rationale behind recommending heavy exercise is simple. A certain level of stress on the body will cause the release of endorphins. Endorphins, you will recall, are the body's natural response to pain. Similar in composition to opiate drugs, they occupy pain receptors and allow the body to tolerate more pain. The positive effect of exercise for endorphin release is somewhat nullified, however, when these same doctors suggest patients take a pain pill *before* exercise. Pain medications depress the body's ability to produce endorphins—again, another vicious cycle. The mechanism that works well in healthy patients once again falls short in fibromyalgics. Exercise is supposed to make patients feel better, but first they must feel well enough to exercise!

The rule should be simple: keep muscular workouts light and within a tolerable discomfort zone, and treat the underlying disease. As patients improve, they can gradually tolerate more exercise, and eventually, more exercise will increase well-being. Suddenly, with effective treatment of fibromyalgia, the vicious circle becomes a road to better health and endurance.

Disability Status—A Raging Controversy

> When it comes to disability determination, anyone who has to prove he or she is ill will be rendered more ill in the proving. When a physician participates in the process it becomes worse than counterproductive, it becomes iatrogenic. At issue is the growing numbers . . . for whom self respect in the workplace is so elusive that the gauntlet of disability determination seems an easier path.
>
> —*Nortin Hadler, M.D.*[32]

The American Medical Association (AMA) declared fibromyalgia a disabling condition more than ten years ago, in

1987. Despite the AMA's straightforward statement, qualifying for these benefits is a major challenge for patients and by extension, for us, their physicians. Unique problems exist because of the subjective nature of complaints and the lack of a diagnostic test capable of proving a patient actually has the disease.

As physicians, we have an obligation to care for our patients. This much is clear. When a patient *says* he is unable to work, it is our duty to help. Yet the absence of an unequivocal diagnostic test relegates us to statements such as: "The patient *states* she is too tired to work, and has headaches every day," or "the patient *says* sitting at her computer makes her back hurt too much to concentrate," or "fibromyalgia is known to cause cognitive problems such as problems with memory and concentration." Insurance companies under pressure to control costs balk and demand proof of disability that meets their criteria. This has locked patients, doctors, lawyers, third-party insurers, and the government in a complicated struggle with no easy solutions.

A physician's letter alone is no longer adequate to qualify for disability. It is only the first step in a long and costly process. Despite a veritable cottage industry on the Internet purporting to teach patients how to obtain benefits, initial denials are routine. Most fibromyalgics end up hiring an attorney for the third and last appeal. It is a dismal situation for the severely incapacitated fibromyalgic, who faces a long and expensive fight. The paperwork, phone interviews and letter-writing are also a burden for the physician.

FMS cases have reached near epidemic proportions in the courts, in U.S. Social Security disability claims, workers' compensation, and accident litigation. As many as 25 percent of U.S. patients with FMS have received some sort of disability or injury compensation.

—*Frederick Wolfe, M.D.*[33]

Insurance companies and governmental agencies are justifiably terrified. Most fibromyalgics are young, and their permanent disability grants are expensive. The sheer number of them is frightening too, especially as the baby boomers push into their forties and fifties. Insurance companies fight back the only way they can, by invoking unread contract clauses and by forcing patients to submit to examination by disability doctors for a second opinion. One long-term disability insurance carrier maintains that fibromyalgia is due to a mental impairment, since there is no definitive test for it. This permits enforcement of the fine-print clause limiting coverage for psychiatric illnesses. Dirty? You bet! But no company is in business to go broke. Other companies take the position that most people are tired and have aches and pains and yet continue to function. On the surface, the latter appears more reasonable, but the end result is the same, benefits are denied. Taxpayers and their legal representatives in the legislature are frightened too. Some states have gone so far as to introduce legislation banning fibromyalgia as a compensable condition, at least in Workers' Compensation cases.

Compassionate physicians should feel that every patient who is reduced to requesting permanent disability status represents a major defeat for medicine. Medicine's victories will come with early diagnosis and physicians who treat the disease instead of symptoms. In younger patients, reversal of their illness is swift and is completed before any thought of disability begins.

As doctors, it is not really our job to think about the system and the financial impact of disability claims. Our concern is more properly whether or not disability is a good long-term treatment for fibromyalgia. We know that remaining active and functional in some capacity is an integral part of self-esteem. Pride in accomplishments is essential to well-being. A job well done, no matter how small, is a good feeling. Long-term disability, like other standard solutions for fibromyalgics, begins a vicious cycle. Patients must first expend a great deal of energy to prove themselves completely unable to be productive. Once the legal battle is won, they must find ways to restore meaning and challenge to everyday life in a way that will not jeopardize an income derived from an inability to perform basic tasks.

Several things are clear: we need assessment criteria that can accurately measure the level of disability in FMS, but more importantly we need to find a way to keep our fibromyalgics as productive as possible. It is an almost inescapable conclusion that we will have to rework the disability system if it is to survive. The answer may lie in more flexible workplace policies mandated by law. More jobs need to be made handicapped-accessible to bolster productivity and self-esteem for everyone.

I know some of the preceding paragraphs will hurt readers who are on disability or in the process of trying to obtain it. But our bottom line is simple. Look back and remember the time when you could have been easily helped if reversal had been available. Would you not have preferred to try it?

I hope that this chapter has answered some questions, but even more I hope that it has underscored our basic tenet: that first of all, we must treat patients with an eye towards getting them well. We should endeavor to make this road as easy as possible. This also means we should be alert to various perils along the way.

> Having a reversal protocol has changed everything. I now see it as a wake-up call and one I have used to empower myself and to heal myself. I feel strong and confident. Without [this] it would be a dreary time of self-blame if not outright depression.
>
> —*M.K., Hawaii*

Chapter 13

❦

Coping with Fibromyalgia:
What Will Help While Guaifenesin
Heals Your Body?

I have been on guai since July 1997—I probably have another two to three years to clear. The past 14 months have not been hell at all. They have been the best 14 months in a long time for me. I know I am healing. I have more energy. I have more stamina. I can do more things, socially, physically, and mentally. So for me, if this is hell—bring it on!

—Linda P., Ohio

In a very real sense, the first day you take guaifenesin is the first day of a new life. You are looking forward to treating the disease itself and to the remission you hope will come in time. You have read other people's stories in this book and maybe you know someone who is getting better taking guaifenesin. Wonderful possibilities are ahead, and for the first time in a long time, you feel hope. Other people got well, and you can, too.

But you are also aware there is more to this treatment than taking a pill. You have read that the treatment is difficult, takes time, and requires both faith and strength. You may also know someone who thinks this treatment is too hard or too complicated. Guaifenesin is after all not for the faint of heart. If it's any consolation, I can tell you straight out that if you've read this far, you've seen a doctor, and you have a bottle of guaifenesin, you don't have to worry too much about this—you are not faint of heart.

What is left now is to think about what you can do while you are waiting for the guaifenesin to do its work. *It's important to mention here that if you are on an adequate dose and you are not blocking it, guaifenesin will work. You do not need to take any other medications. Everything else, as far as we are concerned, is optional.* Since this is the first day of a new life for you, you can use this time to make some simple resolutions to make the road a little easier.

> Nothing could stop me from trying guaifenesin. I was diagnosed in 1988—have tried everything—they all helped to some degree, but not like this. I've had symptoms since at least 1976. I leaped at the chance for this. I have been through so much with this disease over the years—I wanted a chance to get well. The fear of a little more pain was not going to stop me. Besides what guarantee do you have now? My FMS seemed to be getting only worse over the years and here is a chance to change that.
>
> —*Jerri*

🐚 REDUCE STRESS

We all know stress can play a large part in exacerbating the symptoms of FMS or any chronic illness. So as you begin guaifenesin, think about what you can do to make your life a little easier.

First, make sure your doctor has checked you carefully for coexisting conditions. It is important to get other health worries out of the way. If you're on hormone replacement therapy of any kind, be sure that your blood levels are no higher or lower than they should be. If you need to be on the hypoglycemia diet, start it now. The sooner you start it, the sooner you will no longer have blood sugar symptoms to contend with, and if you follow the diet, they'll be completely gone in two months. Difficult at first, the diet will soon become a way of life. Then you will only have to worry about your fibromyalgia.

Think about which medications you want to take and which ones you don't. If you are not overly depressed, understand that your depression is normal because you are ill. It will get better. Think carefully about taking narcotics that you may eventually have trouble discontinuing and which may make you more tired and drowsy. Think about mood-altering drugs and tranquilizers that take away natural highs and lows. You don't want to feel like a zombie, but you may need to make some trade-offs to continue to function. Think about these things now, before your treatment starts. Make sure the doctor you have chosen feels as you do, or will respect your decisions. Having a doctor you feel good about working with will, in itself, lower your stress levels.

Look carefully at the medications and supplements you are taking now. Learn about their side effects and what is known about their safety. If you are uncertain whether or not they are helping you, discuss this with your doctor. This is a new beginning, and it is a good time to take stock of what you are bringing into your new life from your old. If something has not helped you, talk to your doctor about discontinuing it. We have seen many patients clinging to multiple medications they admit have not helped them. They say that they are afraid if they don't take them, they will feel even worse. Examine this thought. If you stop something and you decide it was helping you, you can always start it again. Worrying about what medications you are taking and what they may be doing to you adds stress to your life. Think about how to make your regime as simple as possible.

> I have been doing quite well on my 2400 mg of guai. I still take one Darvocet in the morning and one at bedtime. When comparing this with all the other medications I used to take, I'm doing quite well. So, what have I learned? The road to remission is a journey, not a sprint. The road is not smooth or straight, but it has bumps and twists. Nevertheless, wellness is at the end of it. I'm back on the road, a little smarter than before, and making progress towards my goal of remission in the year 2000.
>
> —*Joel S., Wisconsin*

Stress at Home

First look at the most important place of all—your home. Be sure that those who share your home understand what is going to happen. If you are married or living with another adult, explain the treatment and express your own concerns. You may want to share parts of this book with your family. Explain that you may need their help in the beginning. The hardest thing for most of us to do is to ask for help—we may feel guilty about having asked for so much help in the past—but this time, it's very important. You need your energy to get well.

There are only three secrets for getting help. The first thing is to learn how to ask. Be specific about what you need help with. Don't expect your significant other to know that you want the floor mopped because you are complaining about its being dirty. Don't expect your children to know you want the trash taken all the way out to the curb if you haven't told them exactly where you wanted them to put it. Secondly, if someone is helping you, there's no need to help him. Go away and do something else—rest. Let him do it his way. If it's not exactly the way you would have done it . . . oh well. And, of course, say thank you. Let the other person know, whether it's a child who made you a cup of tea or drew you a picture, or a spouse who cooked dinner and cleaned up afterwards, that you think their effort was wonderful, and how much it means to you that they are helping you to get well.

Everyone in the home should understand what's happening with your health. Keep your explanations simple when you talk to your children. Make sure they understand that you are getting better, but that it will be hard at first, and maybe a little scary, like all new things can be. Make sure they know that there may be some things you just can't do right now, but it isn't your fault or theirs. If you express yourself simply, even very young children can understand and will even learn to think of activities you can share with them. Don't forget that just spending time with them will mean more than anything will. Our time is truly the greatest thing we have to give. Long after toys they had to have are broken and forgotten, children remember the day Mom taught them how to bake cookies.

Board games can substitute for outdoor games when you don't feel well. If your child is old enough, let him read out loud to you, or color with him. On better days, walks together can be refreshing and interesting.

"Lower your standards," may well be the answer for house and garden. "Simplify" is another golden word. This last phrase may well be the words of wisdom for the new millennium— even healthy people have too much to do these days. Everyone, not just fibromyalgics feel stressed out and pressured from all sides. The habits you cultivate during your guaifenesin treatment may even turn out to be beneficial later on.

Use paper plates and eat simple meals. Some people cook a lot when they are feeling well and freeze extra portions for later. Find easy recipes—women's magazines have them, and there are always some on food packages. Crock-Pots—especially in winter—can save you a lot of work, both in preparation time and in cleanup time. And I promise you, kids don't mind grilled cheese sandwiches and soup for dinner. They'd rather have grilled ham and cheese made by a smiling parent than a fancy meal eaten with a stressed-out or exhausted one. Take a deep breath, sit down with your kids while they eat, and talk to them about their day. That alone can make a simple meal special. Microwaves have made life much easier, and if you're on the hypoglycemic diet and the kids aren't, "nuke" something, and sit with them. If your diet won't allow you to break bread with them, eat veggies.

Try not to worry what it looks like behind the refrigerator or under the stove. Remind yourself over and over that there is a time for everything, and this is your time to get well. A spotless house is very low on the list of priorities in life, but health is very high. Remember that, ultimately, good health is the most important thing to have. There will be time enough for everything you want to do when you feel better. Admit that no matter how healthy you may become, your house may never be perfect. After that, it's just a matter of degrees.

There's always the possibility you can pay someone to help with the housework. For some of you the budget just won't allow it, and I don't mean to be insensitive to that fact. But for others, just having someone come in every two weeks or even once a month to do the stove and refrigerator and clean behind things might be possible. Another possibility is to let your kids earn extra money doing housework. They'll probably do it in fits and starts, but even that can provide a break when you're tired.

If your relationship didn't survive the chronic pain and other symptoms of fibromyalgia, there is nothing you can do. You can only consider that you are lucky you learned sooner, rather than later, what the relationship was. You will get well, and when you do, your next choice will be more wise and give you real happiness. Fibromyalgia is a great stressor, but so are many things. If your relationship was not strong enough to survive this illness, it would have eventually faltered anyway.

In the home, as everywhere else, the key is to set reasonable goals for yourself. Think about your priorities and decide what is really important to you. Learn to adapt by, for example, having friends over instead of going out. If you aren't sure you will feel well enough, ask them to understand and bring part of the meal. Learn to recognize situations where you experience less strain and pressure. Simplify and concentrate on what is important. What you are learning now will serve you in good stead all your life.

Have faith, not only in guai, but also in yourself. You would not be trying it if you lacked the one vital trait necessary to heal. That is a determination to see it through. At the end of this road you will find your life again. Is this not worth anything you have to endure? It is similar to the process of birth. At the end of the agony of labor you are gifted with a new life. The pain is forgotten in the joy. The reward is the most precious thing you can possess—your health. If you have your health, you have everything you need. Nothing else compares, as good health enables you to do whatever you desire in life.

> —*Kathy Shuller, Florida*
> *(pain-free, and on my way*
> *out the door)*

Stress in the Workplace

Stress from overwork and anxiety caused by your job can magnify your symptoms and make you feel worse. Don't let work situations weigh you down. If you are able to, spend fewer hours at work.

The problem with that simple advice is that by the time many fibromyalgics begin treatment, they may already be having problems at work. Some have had too many sick days; others have fallen behind or not performed well on days when their fibrofog or fibrogut was bad. If it is feasible, approach your boss and explain what you are doing. Being open and honest up front is always the easiest solution. Hopefully you can come to some agreement to lessen the stress on you as you begin guaifenesin.

If this is not feasible, and you feel that your job would be in jeopardy if you need a few sick days, consider the option of taking some time off at the beginning of treatment. The Family and Medical Leave Act (FLMA) that became law in 1993 may cover you if you work for a company that employs more than fifty people. This law says that if you have a serious health condition that requires continuing treatment by a licensed health care provider, you can take up to twelve weeks unpaid leave to take care of yourself. You will be asked to provide documentation from your doctor and perhaps to give a specific date when you plan to return. This law requires that after your leave is over, you will be restored to the same or an equivalent position with the same pay and benefits. You will have to read this law carefully and talk to your employer, but it may be an option to help you. If your job has a human resource department, you can learn more about your own personal options in detail.

Don't be too frightened or overreact. Despite what you may have heard or read, by far the vast majority of our patients continue working through guaifenesin treatment. Only a few have needed to take a month or two off. We believe that if you can manage it at all, continuing to work is the best option. Remaining productive and as close to your normal routine as possible is always best. If your income is necessary to your family, it may put more stress on you if you try to stop working.

🌸 THINGS YOU CAN DO FOR YOURSELF

Get Enough Sleep

Since one of the main complaints of fibromyalgics is their difficulty sleeping, it is crucial to give your body enough rest. If you had a fitful night of sleep, make it a priority the next day to get additional rest. Lack of sleep on top of the FMS will only exacerbate your symptoms.

When you can manage it, take a little nap. Even if it's just for an hour, a nap can really help. If you are tired at night, go to bed. You can set your alarm clock for half an hour earlier than usual and do some of your unfinished tasks in the morning. You will find they take less time if you face them when you are rested.

Take Warm Baths

Hot or warm baths can soothe your sore muscles and joints and ease the aching pains of FMS. Taking a warm bath before bed can relax you and help you to sleep. Epsom salts can be added to your bath, if you find they help. Be sure to turn down the lights in the bathroom when you bathe.

Understand Your Depression

Along with taking guaifenesin, it's important to take care of your emotional health. Depression can stem from feeling unsuccessful in meeting the standards you have set for yourself at home and at work. Lessening your stress level by coming to terms with your limitations is a good start. Then you can set realistic standards for now. Concentrating on doing your best at what you can do often helps immensely. We have found that for most of our patients, depression begins to lift as their other FMS symptoms start to clear.

Join a Support Group or Start Your Own

> Be careful. There are some groups claiming to be support groups that are actually venting grounds. That is, the people in the group do little more than moan and groan about what a lousy hand life has dealt them. A little venting is good for the soul and the health of everyone. But if the entire discussion is centered on moaning and groaning, it will drag you down into the depths of negativity. *Avoid negative groups.*
> —*Devin J. Starlanyl, M.D.,*
> The Fibromyalgia Advocate[34]

A great deal of comfort can be derived from communication with other fibromyalgics who can offer encouragement and support throughout this process. By connecting with others who understand your pain and have had the same experiences, you feel less isolation and hopelessness. If you have trouble locating a group in your area, try calling the local chapter of the Arthritis Foundation to ask for a list of fibromyalgia support groups. Health care professionals who see a number of fibromyalgic patients may also know of a group. You can also call nearby hospitals to find out whether or not they have a group that meets there.

When you have a list of local groups, pay each a visit to decide if joining it will be a positive addition to your life. A good support group should perform two functions. It should afford its members a needed place to express frustration and other feelings about their illness. Unfortunately, this is where many support groups stop. Meetings seem to consist of sad stories and complaints. It is important to avoid negative groups, since they will drag you down emotionally. The second important function of a support group is that it should strive to improve the quality of your life. It should be a forum for members to help each other with daily tasks. Members can share resources and information about fibromyalgia, good health care providers, and ways to make day-to-day life easier. Some groups even organize car pools, shared child care, or potluck meals. They do just what the name implies—provide support for each other. When one member is not feeling well, others may help out. When another member is lonely, she can call and talk to an empathetic ear. While it's nice to have a guest speaker, you and your group can always attend other groups' meetings for that, and just keep yours more simple.

If no acceptable support group exists in your area, consider starting one of your own. This does not have to be an enormous task. You can start by getting together regularly with a friend or two. You will be amazed at how quickly this will grow into a real group. Work on constructive things: collect simple recipes and helpful tips for improving the quality of your life. At some meetings you can exercise together. You can devise a support system to help each other on bad days.

If you have access to a computer, a world of possibilities exists. Of primary interest to readers of this book is the Internet Guaifenesin Support Group, founded by Tesa Marcon in 1997. To join this group, send an e-mail to the following address: LISTSERV@MAELSTROM.STJOHNS.EDU with the message SUB GUAI-SUPPORT and your full name. You can also subscribe directly from the Guaifenesin Recovery Web site: www.geocities.com/HotSprings/Spa/5252. You will find some other groups and Web sites listed in the Resources section of this book.

Exercise

In this high-tech age, we often forget how simple things can be. Exercise does not require fancy-colored tight-fitting designer togs, and you don't need shiny equipment, hundred-dollar shoes, or a racing bike. You don't need to join a gym, or even buy weights that match your leotards and sweatbands. The sight of well-toned athletes working out with huge weights is intimidating, and exercise like that looks too hard to try. The reality is that very few perfectly healthy people look like that, with perfect bodies, perfect outfits, even, it seems, perfectly placed perspiration. Many more people stay healthy by taking long, peaceful walks with a partner.

There is no doubt that if you can manage it, even modest exercising will make you feel better. Exercise raises the pain threshold through the release of endorphins and has been shown to have a positive effect in ameliorating depression.

If you remember a few simple facts, you can begin to exercise now. Start out modestly. Ambitious starts are the most common cause of defeat. You can begin by walking around the block or working with a gentle exercise video on your living room floor. There are some exercise tapes designed for fibromyalgics, which you can find in the Resources section of this book. You will learn from them to recognize and honor your own tolerance levels.

Exercise should never be done when your muscles are cold or tired. Do some mild stretching before you begin. Devin Starlanyl, M.D., in her book, *The Fibromyalgia Advocate*, offers an excellent rule of thumb for designing an exercise program:

If mild soreness disappears after the first day, you can repeat it on the second day. If it persists to the second day, postpone any exercise until the third day. If soreness persists on the third day, your exercise routine must be changed. This rule of thumb is true for any treatment, such as massage or electrical stimulation.[35]

For those who prefer organized exercise programs, the Arthritis Foundation can usually direct you to some that will meet your needs. Their Aquatic Program can be especially helpful, and you can ask them for brochures about it. It is a program of exercises done in warm water designed for those with limited mobility. There are many other programs that offer exercise classes as well, so be sure to check around.

Yoga, tai chi, and other disciplines all have their advocates in our practice. Exercise programs are as individual as everything else in fibromyalgia is, and we encourage our patients to keep trying until they find an exercise regimen they like. The one consensus is that if you force yourself to do some exercise and are careful not to overdo it, you will feel better.

After about three months on the guai I decided to try exercising on my stationary bike again. . . . I have found that when I am really hurting, if I ride the bike for at least 15 minutes the pain begins to ease up. It is really hard to convince myself to get started when it hurts to even walk, let alone really exercise. But the benefits are worth it. Evenings are my worst times and I find that if I ride my bike for about 30 minutes just before bedtime, I get rid of a lot of my pain and become very relaxed. This promotes a good sleep that often leads to a better day afterward.

—*Marilyn J., North Carolina*

Massage and Body Work

Body work is done by practitioners who use touch and physical contact for healing. Practically no one discounts the power of human contact in promoting well-being. A visit to a trained massage therapist who understands fibromyalgia for a gentle massage can ease the pain in your muscles, and more. There is something intrinsically comforting about being touched.

Avoid deep-tissue work and stay away from Rolfing—these techniques will increase your pain. The wrong kind of massage can be painful at the time and for days afterwards. Always make sure the practitioner you visit is knowledgeable about fibromyalgia. You can ask if he has a brochure or printed material about his technique and how it applies to your condition. Ask your doctor and support group for recommendations if you need a place to start.

I have had patients tell me that acupuncture relieves their pain quite well. Some newer medical papers support this idea, although we have had other patients who have not found it particularly beneficial. Chiropractors who specialize in fibromyalgia are also a good resource; we have had many patients get real help from them.

A bodywork technique we have seen to benefit patients is known as the Feldenkrais Method. In a series of lessons, patients are taught how to integrate their body movements so that they function with less effort and pain. The movements are slow and gentle, and the individual instruction and retraining are helpful. Similar disciplines such as the Alexander Technique and the Bowen Therapy may also be tried.

After any kind of treatment, plan on getting some rest. Your body has been working hard. You may find when you get home that a warm bath will make you feel better.

There is no question that body work and massage therapies are expensive. Not every patient has insurance, and not every insurance company will cover even basic chiropractic care. Most regard massage as a luxury. Patients should always remember that these therapies will, at best, only make them feel more comfortable while the guaifenesin does its work. They are not a necessary part of healing.

There are colleges of massage therapy that charge much smaller fees than do the professionals. I had my second visit at my local school and I am still sold on the idea. I even took my sister-in-laws and the four of us got in on a two-for-one special: $10 a person! They are now sold on the idea too. One important note: although there may be one main address for the school, there are often additional locations of that school in different cities in your state. Take Utah for example— there is one school but it has three different locations throughout the state. Contact the schools in your state for more information on additional locations.

—*Sharon H., Utah*

✤ DO SOMETHING YOU LOVE EVERY DAY

I used to put "baking cookies with my son" on my list almost every week because we would talk while we were cooking, and he loved that. I would tell him about when I was a little girl and how I used to watch my mother bake, and it made me happy to remember good things. If I did nothing else at all that day, at least I did that. I made a vow not to flog myself for what I could not do—not to sit and watch other mothers running after their kids and beat myself up anymore. Instead I focused on the tasks I had made for myself . . . and counted myself lucky when I could do them.

—*C.P., Marina del Rey, CA*

The worst thing to do for your own mental health is to stop doing the things that are important to *you*. That is the quickest way to lose hope, the quickest way to feel defeated, as if you are sinking into a life that has little pleasure left. You must stay in touch with yourself and who you were before your disease took over your life. This is hard to do—very hard. As our disease progressed, most of us stopped doing just about everything we enjoyed to save our strength for the endless list of things we felt we had to do. That was natural. But now, with guaifenesin, we are beginning again. In simplifying our lives, we can recover some of the things we lost.

I found that there were activities I had stopped doing long ago, such as playing the piano and sewing, that really make me feel good. . . . If I am sad or stressed, perhaps experiencing early warning signs of an approaching flare, I make sure to spend some time involved in such an activity. It makes me feel better and my life feels enriched.

—*Mary Ellen Copeland, coauthor,* Fibromyalgia & Chronic Myofascial Pain Syndrome[36]

Start by deciding what makes you feel good and what you love. Time for your partner, time for your children, of course, but then . . . what do *you* love to do? What makes *you* feel better when you do it? Is it working in the garden, painting with watercolors, reading a book, or doing a crossword puzzle? Do you like taking a slow, quiet walk in the evening, or like to sit outside in the morning sun and have a cup of tea? What can you think of that makes you feel good when you do it, so good that sometimes when you do it you lose track of time?

Start there. Make a list of those things and of other things that are important to you. If it is important to watch your son's soccer games, put it on the list. You may enjoy watching your child sitting in the park during the last days of Indian summer when the evenings are golden. If logging onto a newsgroup and supporting others makes you feel good, put that on the list too.

After you finish the first list, list the days of the week. On each day note down one simple task, such as changing the sheets on the bed or cleaning out the car, and one thing you love to do, like working in the garden for an hour. Then, on that day, make sure you do those two things. If you learn to do this, you will keep in touch with yourself. When you are alone or around other people you will feel better. Life itself will seem richer and more meaningful. You will learn things you had forgotten about yourself. This confidence will help you in your interactions with doctors, with friends, and with family. It will help you to focus on getting well.

Whatever your life has in store, it will help to know who you are and what is really important to you. The key to success is to know what you love to do, and to find a way to do it. Guaifenesin will give you back your health, but only you can reclaim your own life.

❦

The Authors' Last Word

If you have read this far from beginning to end, despite your fibrofog, pain, and fatigue, I am impressed. As I was writing these pages, I wondered how to end this book. I also wondered how long some of you would bear with me. I have offered you reversing cycles of fatigue, cognitive blurs, and added pain. I have taken away your favorite herbs, your cosmetics, and for some of you, chocolate, potatoes, pasta, bread, and your favorite desserts. Yet here you are.

Luckily, most physicians are now able to make the diagnosis of fibromyalgia, and we make weekly additions to our list of doctors who are willing to prescribe guaifenesin to treat it. With some diligence and persistence you should be able to find a physician to work with you. You must remember, though, that it is not fair to expect doctors to do more than prescribe your medicine, monitor your progress, and warn you about salicylates. Avoiding salicylates will be your responsibility. Be prepared to do your own legwork.

It is less likely that you will find a doctor who will accept the method I have described for making the diagnosis of hypoglycemia. The forty percent of you who suffer from carbohydrate intolerance and fibromyalgia, our poor fibroglycemics, will need to recognize this syndrome on your own and follow the appropriate diet. After all, you do not need a doctor to tell you that eating too many carbohydrates does not agree with you. Once you discover that the diet makes you feel better, it is your responsibility to stay on it.

If you have ongoing hypoglycemia, the treatment is black and white. We have listed what you can eat and drink. It is a straightforward diet that has worked for my patients for more than thirty years, and all you need is discipline for a few months. You *can* do it. Approach it with a positive attitude because it was designed to help you feel better.

A few of you are wondering: "How can I possibly do this?" Unfortunately, you are not alone. We have grown accustomed to hearing from those who just can't do it. Yet the majority of you will embrace the procedure and follow the protocol. You who have not given up on life will be rewarded. But you must be willing to pay the toll to drive on the road back—the one that ends with restoration of your health.

For those with fibromyalgia, the initial search for salicylates which block guaifenesin demands time and patience. Once it has been completed, all that remains is to closely guard against errors when replacing products. The treatment is simple enough. Take the guaifenesin, find your dose, and then give it time to work. The intensity of the reversal cycles will vary for each of you. When it seems difficult, it will help to remember a few facts:

- You were not well before you started, and your fibromyalgia was actually getting worse before you began our treatment.

- You will feel worse at first, but since guaifenesin has no significant side effects, more intense cycles mean the drug is working.

- It took time to develop fibromyalgia. It will take less time to get rid of it, but it will still take time.

- Your first good hours will tell you that your body is capable of recovery.

- There is happiness ahead. To me, happiness means freedom from pain—mental and physical.

We who have conquered the disease owe something to those who are still sick. As wonderful as it is to feel well, there will remain an emptiness if we are up on the victory stand without the rest of you. I hope this book will become like a chain letter. As each of you becomes well, you, in turn, will be in debt. You can only repay this debt by helping others who are still looking for the way to good health. We must not give up as long as there are still those who are suffering as we once did.

—R. Paul St. Amand, M.D.
Claudia Craig Marek

Appendix 1:
One Thousand of the Most Common Natural Salicylates to Avoid

Acacia
Acerola
Achillea
Acorns
Adder's tongue
Adonis vernalis
Agar
Agave lechuguilla
Agrimony (Agrimonia)
Ajaga
Alehoof
Alfalfa
Algae
Algin
Allspice
Almond (oil)
Aloe (vera)
Alpine cranberry
Althea root
Alum
Amantilla
Amaranth (Amaranthus)
Amber

Ambrette seed
American centaury
American desert herb
American hellebore
American ivy
American mountain ash
American saffron
Amica
Amyris
Anemone
Anethole
Angelica
Angostura bark
Anise (aniseed)
Annedda pychogenol
Apple (blossom)
Apricot
Arbutus extract
Arnica
Aromatic bitters
Arrowroot
Artemisia annua
Artichoke extract

Arum
Asarum
Asclepias
Ash
Asparagus (root)
Aspen
Astragalus
Atlas cedarwood
Avens
Avocado
Babassu
Balm (mint, lemon balm)
Balm of Gilead extract
Balsam (mecca, oregon, peru, tolu, etc.)
Bamboo
Banana
Baneberry
Baptisia
Barberry
Bardane (Bardana)
Barley grass
Basil
Bay laurel
Bay leaf
Bayberry
Bean
Bearberry
Bearded darnel
Bear's garlic
Bedstraw
Bee balm extract
Bee pollen

Beech
Beechdrop
Beetroot
Belladonna
Bennet's root
Berberis
Bergamot
Betony
Betula
Bi yan pian
Bilberry complex/extract
Bilva
Birch
Bird's tongue
Birthroot
Birthwort
Bisabol (or bisabolol)
Bistort
Bitter almond
Bitter cherry
Bitter orange
Bitterroot
Bitterstick
Black alder
Black birch
Black cohosh
Black currant
Black haw (bark)
Black mustard
Black pepper
Black root
Black thistle
Black walnut

Blackberry

Blackwort

Bladder wrack

Blazing star

Blessed thistle

Blind nettle

Blood root

Blue cohosh

Blue flag

Blue-green algae

Blue gum eucalyptus

Blue vervain

Blueberry leaves

Bogbean

Bois de rose (oil)

Boldo leaf

Boneset

Borage (oil)

Borneol

Boronia

Boswellia

Bougainvillea

Bourtree

Boxwood

Brahami

Bran

Brassica

Brazilian guarana

Brazilwood

Brier hip

Brigham tea

Broad-leaved peppermint
    eucalyptus

Brooklime

Broom oil

Bryony (Byronia)

Buchu

Buckbean

Buckthorn

Buckwheat

Bugle weed

Bugloss (extract)

Burdock (root, extract)

Butchers' broom

Butterbur

Buttercup

Butterfly weed

Butternut (root, bark)

Cabbage (extract)

Cabbage rose

Cabreuva

Cacao

Cactus (Cactus grandiflorus)

Cade

Cajeput

Calamintha

Calamus

Calendula

California poppy

Calophyllum (oil)

Camellia (oil)

Camphor

Canada root

Canadian balsam

Canaga

Candleberry

Candlenut tree

Candock

Canenula

Cannabis

Canola oil

Capers

Capsicum

Caraway

Cardemom

Carline thistle

Carnation

Carnauba (wax okay)

Carrot (oil, seed)

Cascara sagrada

Cascarilla bark

Cashew nut (oil)

Cassia

Castor (bean, oil)

Catechu

Catharanthus

Catnip

Cat's Claw

Catuaba

Cayenne

Ceanothus (extract)

Cedar

Celandine (extract)

Celery (seed)

Centaury (Centaurea)

Chamomile (Camomile)

Chaparral (extract)

Chaste tree

Cherimoya

Cherry (bark, pit, pit oil)

Chervil

Chestnut

Chia (oil)

Chickory

Chickweed

Chili

Chimaphila

China bark

Chinese angelica (root)

Chinese hibiscus

Chinese magnolia

Chinese tea

Chives

Chrysanthemum

Chuan xin lian

Cilantro

Cinchona

Cinnamon

Cinquefoil

Citronella

Citrus (seed, seed extract)

Clary sage

Cleavers (cleaverwort)

Clematis extract

Clove

Clover

Club moss

Cocoa

Coconut

Cohosh (root)

Colchicum

Cola (nuts, seeds)

Colombo
Coltsfoot
Columbine
Comfrey
Condurango (extract)
Coneflower
Copaiba balsam
Copal
Coral root
Coriander
Corn mint
Cornflower
Cornsilk
Corydalis
Costus
Cottonseed (oil)
Couch grass (root, root extract)
Coumarin
Cowslip
Cramp bark
Cranberry
Crane's bill (extract)
Crataegus
Crocus
Cubeb
Cucumber
Cudweed (extract)
Culver's root
Cumin
Curcumin
Curled dock
Currant
Curry

Cyclamen
Cyperus
Cypress
Daisy
Damask rose
Damiana
Dandelion (leaf, root)
Date
Davana (oil)
Deer tongue
Delphinium
Desert tea
Devil's claw
Dill
Dinkum (oil)
Dock
Dog poison
Dogbane (Dogsbane)
Dog's mercury
Dogtooth violet
Dogwood
Dong quai
Drosera
Dulcamara (extract)
Dwarf pine
Dyer's broom
Easter rose
Echinacea
Elder
Elderflower
Elderberry
Elecampane
Elemi

Eleuthero
Elm bark
Elymus
English ivy
English oak extract
English walnut
Ephedra
Epimedium
Ergot
Erigeron (oil)
Escin
Esculin
Estragon (oil)
Eucalyptus
Euphorbia
Euphrasia (Euphrasy)
European ash
European centaury
European vervain
Evening primrose (oil)
Everlasting
Exotic basil
Eyebright
Fava bean
Fennel
Fenugreek (Foenugreek) (seed)
Fern
Ferula
Feverfew
Feverweed
Feverwort
Field poppy
Fig

Figwort
Fir needle oil
Flavonoids
Flax (seed, oil)
Flowering spurge
Fo-ti
Foxglove
Frankincense
Fraxinella
French basil
Fringe tree
Fumitory
Galangal
Galbanum
Galega
Galium aparine
Gallweed
Gan mo ling
Garden balsam
Garden spurge
Garden thyme
Garden violet
Gardenia
Garlic
Gay gee
Gentian root
Geraniol
Geranium
German chamomile
Germander
Ginger
Ginkgo biloba
Ginseng

Goat weed
Goat's rue
Goldenrod
Goldenseal
Goldthread
Gotu Kola
Gourd
Grape leaf
Grapefruit
Grapeseed
Gravel root
Great burnet
Great periwinkle
Green bean
Green tea
Grindelia
Ground ivy
Groundsel
Guaiacwood
Guar gum
Guarana
Guava
Gum karaya
Gum plant
Hamamelis
Hawaiian white ginger
Hawkweed
Hawthorne (Hawthorne berry)
Hay maids
Hayflower
Hazel
Heartsease
Heather

Hedge bindweed
Hedge hyssop
Hedge mustard
Hedge parsley
Helichrysum
Heliotrope
Hellebore
Hemlock spruce
Hemp (Hemp agrimony,
    Hemp nettle)
Henbane
Henna
Hepatica
Herb Robert
Hesperidin
Hibiscus
Holly
Hollyhock
Holy thistle
Honey
Honeydew melon
Honeysuckle
Hops
Horehound
Horse chestnut
Horse nettle
Horsemint (oil)
Horseradish
Horsetail
Horseweed
Hound's-tongue
Houseleek
Huang qi

Huckleberry (leaf)
Hyacinth
Hybrid safflower
Hydrangea
Hydrocotyl
Hydrophilia
Hypericum
Hyssop
Iceland moss
Immortelle
Impatiens
Imperial masterwort
Indian cress
Indian hemp
Indian poke
Indian turnip
Indigo
Ipecac
Irish moss
Ironweed
Ivy
Jaborandi
Jalap
Jamaica dogwood
Jambul
Japanese turf lily
Jasmine
Java jute
Jesuit's tea
Jewelweed
Jimson weed
Johnny-jump-up
Jojoba

Jonquil
Judas tree
Jujube
Juniper
Kangaroo paw
Kava kava
Kawa
Kelp
Khus-khus
Kidney bean
Kidney vetch
Kino
Kiwi
Klamath weed
Knee holy
Knotgrass
Knotted figwort
Knotweed
Ko ken
Kola (Kola nut)
Kousso
Krameria
Kudzu root
Kuikui (nut, nut oil)
Labdanum
Labrador tea
Lad's love
Lady's mantle
Lady's slipper
Lady's thistle
Lappa
Larch
Larkspur

Laurel leaf
Lavandin
Lavender
Leek
Lemon
Lemon balm
Lemon verbena
Lemongrass
Lemon-scented eucalyptus
Lentil
Lesquerella
Lettuce
Levant styrax
Lichen
Licorice (licorice root)
Lilac
Liliaceae
Lily (Lily of the valley)
Lime
Linaloe
Linalool
Linden
Linseed
Lion's foot
Litsea cubeba
Liverwort
Lobelia
Locust bean
Longleaf pine
Loose strife, purple
Loquat
Lotus
Lovage

Lungwort
Lupin
Lycii
Lycopodium
Ma hsing chih ke pien
Macadamia
Madder
Magnolia
Ma huang
Maiden hair fern
Maitake mushroom
Mallow
Malva
Mandarin (mandarin orange)
Mandrake
Mango
Marigold
Marijuana
Marine extracts
Maritime pine extract
Marjoram
Maroc chamomile
Marsh tea
Marshmallow root
Masterwort
Mastic
Mate
Matico
Matricaria
Meadow saffron
Meadowfoam (Meadowfoam seed)
Meadowsweet

Meliae seeds
Melilotus
Melissa
Mentha (Aquatica, Piperita, etc.)
Mexican damiana
Mezereon
Milfoil
Milk thistle
Milk-purslane
Milkweed
Milkwort
Millet
Mimosa
Mint
Mistletoe
Monarda
Monkshood
Moringa
Mormon tea
Mortierella
Moss spores
Mother of thyme
Motherwort
Mountain ash berries
Mountain laurel
Mountain maple
Mouse ear
Mugwort
Muira puama
Mulberry
Mullein leaf
Mushroom

Musk rose
Musk-mallow
Muskmelon
Mustard
Myrcia
Myrrh
Myrtle
Narcissus
Nasturtium
Neem tree
Nenuphar
Nerve root
Nettles
New Jersey tea
Niaouli
Nicotana
Nightshade
Nutmeg
Oak bark
Oakmoss
Oat flower (oat root, oat straw)
Oleander
Olive (olive oil)
Onion
Opopanax
Orange (orange blossom, orange oil)
Orchid
Oregano (seed, oil)
Oregon grape (root)
Origanum (oil)
Orris
Osha

Oswego tea
Pacific yew
Palm oil (palm kernel oil)
Palmarosa
Panama bark
Pansy
Papaya
Paprika
Paraguay tea
Parsley
Pasque flower
Passiflora or Passion flower
Patchouli
Pau d'arco
Pawpaw
Pea
Peach (Peach kernel oil)
Peanut
Pear
Pectin
Pennyroyal
Pennywort
Peony
Pepper (oil, black, red, green)
Peppermint (Peppermint oil)
Periwinkle
Persic (oil)
Peru balsam
Peruvian bark
Petitgrain
Pettier
Petty spurge
Peyote

Pichi
Pilewort
Pimenta leaf
Pimpernel
Pine (bark, cone, pycnogenol,
    needle oil)
Pineapple
Pinkroot
Pinus pulmilio
Pinyon pine
Pipissewa
Pitcher plant
Plantago (seed)
Plantain
Pleurisy (root)
Plum
Podophyllum
Poison hemlock
Pokeroot
Pokeweed
Pollen
Pomegranate
Poplar
Poppy
Pot marigold
Potato
Prickly ash (bark)
Pride of China
Primrose
Primula
Privet
Prosperity
Psoralea

Pueraria
Pukeweed
Pumpkin
Purging cassia
Pycnogenol
Quassia
Queen-of-the-meadow
Queen's delight
Quercus
Quillaja (bark)
Quillay (bark)
Quince (seed)
Quinine
Quinoa (extract)
Radish
Ragged cup
Ragwort
Raisin (seed, oil)
Rapeseed (oil)
Raspberry (juice, leaf)
Rattlesnake plantain
Rauwolfia (extract)
Raw honey
Red clover
Red eyebright
Red pepper
Red pimpernel
Red raspberry leaf
Red root
Red sandalwood
Red sedge
Rehmannia
Reishi mushroom

Restharrow (extract)
Rhatany
Rhodinol
Rhododendron
Rhubarb (root)
Rock-rose
Roman chamomile
Rosa californica
Rosa centifolia
Rosa damascena
Rosa eglanteria
Rosa gallica
Rosa laevigata
Rosa roxburghi
Rose (leaves, extract, oil,
    hips—vitamin C source)
Rose bengal
Rose bulgarian
Rose geranium
Rosemary
Rosewood
Rowan
Royal jelly
Rue
Rutin
Sabal
Safflower (oil)
Saffron crocus
Safrole
Sage
Sagebrush
Salicaria
Sambucus

Sandalwood

Sanicle

Santolina

Sarsaparilla (root)

Sassafras

Savine

Savory

Saw palmetto

Shavegrass

Schinus molle

Schisandra

Scotch broom

Scotch pine

Scullcap

Scurvy grass

Sea holly

Seaweed

Sedge root

Senega snakeroot

Senna

Septfoil

Sesame seed oil

Seven barks

Shanka puspi

Shave grass

Sheep sorrel

Shepherd's purse

Shield fern extract

Shinleaf

Shitake mushroom

Shunis

Silver fir needle

Silymarin

Skullcap

Skunk cabbage

Slippery elm bark

Snakeroot

Snapdragon

Soapberry extract

Soapwort extract

Solomon's seal

Sorbus extract

Sorrel extract

Southern wood

Spanish broom

Spanish moss

Spanish oregano

Spanish sage

Spearmint

Speedwell

Spike lavender

Spikenard

Spinach (extract)

Spiraea (extract)

Spirulina

Spotted cranebill

Spotted hemlock (root, extract)

Spruce (oil)

Spurge

Squaw vine

Squill

St. Bartholomew's tea

St. Benedict thistle

St. John's wort

Star anise

Star grass

Stevia (used as an herbal medication, not as a sweetener)
Sticklewort
Stiff gentian
Stillingia
Stoneflower
Stoneroot
Storax
Storksbill
Stramonium
Strawberry
Strawflower
Strophanthus
Strychnos
Sumac
Summer savory
Sundew
Sunflower (seed, oil)
Sweet almond oil
Sweet balm
Sweet bay (oil)
Sweet birch
Sweet cicely
Sweet clover
Sweet fern
Sweet flag
Sweet grass
Sweet gum
Sweet marjoram
Sweet orange
Sweet violet
Swertia
Sycamore maple

Tacamahac
Tagetes
Tall oil
Tamarack
Tamarind
Tangerine (oil)
Tang kuei
Tansy
Taro
Tarragon
Tea
Tea tree
Texas cedarwood
Thistle
Thoroughwort
Thuja
Thunder vine
Thyme
Tiare flower
Tilia
Toad flax
Tobacco
Tolu balsam
Tomato (extract)
Tonka
Tormentil
Trailing arbutus
Tree moss
True lavender
Tuberose
Tulips
Tun-hoof
Turkey corn

Turkey rhubarb
Turkey-red oil
Turmeric
Turnip extract
Turtlebloom
Twin leaf
Ultra Primrose
Unicorn root
Uva-ursi
Vacha
Valerian root
Vanilla
Veratrum
Verbena
Veronica
Vervain
Vetiver
Violet
Virginia snakeroot
Virginian cedarwood
Virgin's bower
Viscum
Vitex
Wafer ash
Wahoo
Walnut (extract, leaves, shell oil)
Water avens
Water chestnut
Water eryngo
Water lily
Water pimpernel
Watercress

Watermelon
Wax berry
Wax myrtle
West Indian bay
Wheat germ
White birch
White cedar leaf oil
White ginger
White mustard
White nettle
White oak bark
White pine
White pond lily
White poplar
White sage
White weed
White willow bark
Wild agrimony extract
Wild black cherry
Wild carrot
Wild cherry bark
Wild clover
Wild daisy
Wild ginger
Wild hyssop
Wild indigo root
Wild jalap
Wild marjoram
Wild mint
Wild Oregon grape
Wild sarsaparilla
Wild strawberry
Wild thyme

Wild yam (root)
Willow bark
Willow leaf
Winter savory
Wintergreen
Wisteria
Witch grass
Witch hazel
Woad
Wood betony
Wood sorrel
Woodruff
Wormseed
Wormwood
Woundwort
Yam
Yara yara

Yarrow
Yellow curled dock
Yellow dock root
Yellow gengian
Yellow goatsbeard
Yellow jessamine
Yellow melilot
Yellow parilla
Yellow toadflax
Yerba santa
Yerbamate
Yew
Yin qiao
Ylang ylang
Yohimbe (Yohimbine bark)
Yucca

Appendix 2: Technical Appendix

 FIBROMYALGIA AND HYPOGLYCEMIA:
REVERSAL BY TREATMENT AND THEORY
OF CAUSE

In order to explain my theory of this dysenergism—which I believe is a more appropriate name for the illness we commonly call fibromyalgia—I will make use of currently accepted biochemistry, and interject my own thoughts. In the more than forty years since I began working with fibromyalgia, I have tried to understand its pathochemistry and the reason for my treatment's success. In the Preface of this book I stated that I am as certain about the efficacy of treatment as I am that errors will be found in my theory. I sincerely expect erudite additions and deletions by clinicians. I reserve my most hopeful praise, in advance, for the geneticists and biochemists who will eventually define the pathology of fibromyalgia. I ask that we try to add to our knowledge and display mutual respect. We are all striving to provide answers to a miserable disease that ruins many lives.

Dysenergism—or lack of adequate energy—is common to both fibromyalgia and hypoglycemia. In the text of this book, I explained that a large percentage of our fibromyalgic patients suffer from hypoglycemia, as that term should be newly defined. The frequent interweaving of these two conditions mandates my discussing them together, even though both may exist independently. Each of these metabolic misadventures greatly augments the problems caused by the other. I have coined the word "fibroglycemia" to designate those who suffer from both entities.

Biologists know that nature's design is simple: one is born, gets nourishment, grows to maturity, procreates, nurtures the young to self-sufficiency, and is disposed of. All other purposes are human affectations adding charm to life or to the basic design. Our amusements—enjoying delectable repasts, television viewing, selecting wines, traveling, shopping for fashions, and maintaining luxurious homes—only fill the time gaps available when we are not busy satisfying our ingrained, primordial needs.

We require abundant energy formation from our chemical factories, the mitochondria, simply to serve our inborn, biological mandates. In addition, we expend a great deal of effort to energize our social whims and, as a consequence, often allow insufficient time for normal repair. Our construct is such that we take the easy way out, and use carbohydrate fuels as short-cuts for energy production and quick starts for our activities. In lieu of using healthier fuels, this approach is successful for most, even though it presents potential problems. Sugars and starches provide rapid-fire energy sparks, but in some patients these foods cause erratic insulin spikes that are poorly counter-regulated. These insulin spurts do not permit a smooth interplay between energy utilization and storage. Glucose and insulin soar in tandem and guarantee that, within a few hours, there will be a precipitous drop in blood sugar. For the hypoglycemia-prone, repeated insulin release and falling blood sugar have serious consequences. Even without hypoglycemia, insulin invokes progressive, subliminal damage. Medical literature is replete with articles describing the deleterious effects of insulin excesses on hypertension, serum lipids, obesity, arteriosclerosis (syndrome X), the immune system, and so forth.

I assume that those who delve into this chapter have read my descriptions of fibromyalgia, hypoglycemia, and their interplay, even though they were written for the lay reader. There I explain how I had found success treating fibromyalgia with uricosuric agents, but that each of these had certain side effects. Those who reacted adversely to all of them were left without options. I had no other solutions until I chanced upon an article about the uricosuric effect of guaifenesin, a mucolytic agent. Guaifenesin is minimally uricosuric, but is, without a doubt, the most potent and safest weapon I have found for reversing fibromyalgia.

It seems obvious to me that there is a multigenetic cause of fibromyalgia. We have treated several young children but we have also seen the illness develop later in life, even in the elderly. Depending upon the degree of genetic influence, variable levels of trauma can precipitate fibromyalgia in patients. I have no doubt that fibromyalgia is an inherited disease that involves more than one or two genes. It is obvious that a spectrum of possibilities exist. In those who have only minor defects in the amino acid sequences of the genes responsible, fibromyalgia may never fully manifest. These are individuals who will suffer transient fibromyalgic symptoms when they are sufficiently traumatized by an accident, surgery, serious infection, or prolonged stress. These situations demand immediate, large bursts of energy, in excess of the generating capacity. A limited ability to produce ATP does not allow the luxury of florid energy expenditures. Mildly affected patients can eventually purge the damage-induced, metabolic debris within a very variable time frame, determined by their own mitochondrial prowess. They will suffer an ATP shortage only when repairs are required which overtax their generating capacities. For those with a more dominant gene, minor stresses or injuries may seem to precipitate chronic fibromyalgia. It is clear that genetically, they were destined to develop the disease eventually. It is confusing to physicians who witness posttraumatic symptoms of fibromyalgia because they appear to be part of the general damage brought on by the stress.

My relatively long career in medicine has given me the time to examine, on many occasions, three generations of family members. I am impressed by the probability that fibromyalgia is a harbinger of osteoarthritis. Most osteoarthritics I have questioned and mapped have had the same symptoms and findings as their fibromyalgic siblings or progeny. This does not include patients with traumatic osteoarthritis. The duration of the disease determines the extent of involvement. If fibromyalgia is allowed to progress unchecked, it is my experience that it will eventually lead to joint damage, contrary to current teaching.

All the agents we have used successfully have increased proximal renal tubular excretion of urates. They are not known to have any other mutual effects on the body. When used for gout, each is blocked by even tiny amounts of salicylate. This chemical obstruction takes place at the proximal tubular level. The singular success of guaifenesin and the other totally disparate molecules in treating fibromyalgia allows me to conclude that it is a retention disease like gout. It is also logical to suspect a renal tubular defect as the culprit. Whatever substance is retained demonstrates a far greater invasiveness and ability to disperse itself throughout the body than do urates. The elimination of anions is normally orchestrated with great precision, depending on metabolic needs. It appears that the genetic aberration that causes fibromyalgia encodes for a defective receptor, enzyme, ion channel, chemical signaling, or carrier protein.

Medical personnel are well aware that laboratory tests show no diagnostic changes. The body mounts no inflammatory response against what it perceives as normal body constituents. We can extrapolate from gout and its negatively charged urate that an anion is the likely causative agent of fibromyalgia. Which anion could be retained in sufficient quantity to impede energy formation and yet escape detection?

I have described the effects of guaifenesin and the uricosuric agents on dental calculus and fingernail growth. All may induce chipping or lysing of calculus and gradually reverse the abnormal breakage of fingernails. Tartar and fingernails are both composed largely of calcium phosphate. These observations imply some effect of our various medications on the metabolism of one or the other of these ions. But which one?

An anion capable of blocking energy formation would have to be one that is normally involved in the production of ATP. Inorganic phosphate is the likely suspect. In support of this, we measured urinary excretion of phosphates in the subsequent forty-eight hours after instigating treatment with either probenecid or guaifenesin. Both uricosuric agents and guaifenesin seem to have a fairly strong phosphaturic effect. A sixty percent increase over baseline was observed in phosphate excretion, as well as about one half of that amount in increased oxalate and calcium. Biochemists are finding that anions are as closely regulated as are cations. A disturbance in phosphate metabolism is my choice for the systemwide ravages of fibromyalgia. It is my premise that excess phosphate accumulated due to a genetic defect will eventually have deleterious effects.

Energy changes can be depicted by the formula:

$$\Delta G = \frac{ATP}{ADP + Pi}$$

(ΔG = energy change)
(Pi=inorganic phosphate)

Some years ago, Bengtsson and Henriksson biopsied trapezial lesions in fibromyalgics and reported deviations from normal controls. They found decreases in seventeen percent in ATP and tweny-one percent in phosphocreatine, the reservoir for high-energy phosphates. They also pointed out that the involved fibers were even more severely affected than the above percentages indicate because specimens were diluted by normal fibers of adjacent tissue.[37] Control biopsies from healthy individuals, when similarly analyzed, showed like changes in only a few fibers. Significantly, they observed that not all fibers within a given specimen are affected. This confirms that there is no innate defect in the muscle itself. It is more likely that a chemical imbalance occurs as something enters the affected mitochondria and causes faulty ATP formation.

This excellent study supports the theory of defective ATP formation, as have researchers such as Dr. Robert Bennett.

> Mechanical forces during muscular contraction, particularly eccentric contraction, cause disruption of muscle fibers and disturb the permeability of the sarcolemmal membrane. This results in a net influx of calcium ions and an efflux of potassium ions. High concentrations of calcium in muscle cells cause a state of persistent contraction (without electromyographic activity); this utilizes ATP/phosphorylcreatine, thus depleting energy stores.[38]

There is only one way to keep a muscle contracted: free ionic calcium in the sarcoplasm. It is also, somewhat ironically, the mechanism of rigor mortis.

I believe that due to an inherited defect, proximal renal tubules are unable to excrete the exact amount of phosphate ions required for systemic balance. While inexorable retention may begin at birth, the ion can be buffered for a variable number of years by dispersal throughout many tissues, especially bones. The number of affected genes determines the time of symptom onset and the severity of symptoms.

Inorganic phosphate has two negative charges and, in my scheme, is buffered mainly by the two positive charges of calcium that must also enter cells, probably to a lesser excess. Calcium is not normally allowed free range within the sarcoplasm or cytosol. In nearly all cells it is the final messenger that forces compliance with whatever action has been requested by the initial stimulus. This call to action will continue until calcium is either extruded from the cell or returned into storage within the endoplasmic reticulum. Calcium is purged from the cytosol by ATP-driven pumps. It has been reported that up to forty-five percent of the body's ATP is utilized for this one activity. The fibromyalgic's high cytosolic calcium increases metabolism in all cells and makes demands on an already inadequate ATP availability. Affected cells are driven to exhaustion but continue their enfeebled attempt to respond to the calcium prodding. The system must protect itself from cell death—apoptosis. It obviously succeeds at this, since no permanent damage occurs in fibromyalgia until much later, when calcium phosphate crystals form in joints, the last of the body's relatively safe storage sites.

It makes sense that fibromyalgia is an overwork syndrome caused by cells and systems pushed into continuing activity by the presence of cytosolic calcium. But the true villain is phosphate that enters the mitochondrial matrix to excess and hinders ATP formation. How does phosphate alter mitochondrial function sufficiently to interfere with such a fundamental cellular need?

The cellular membrane protects its interior from uncontrolled surges of ions and molecules. This is accomplished by the cell's electrical potential, its many receptors, channels, carrier proteins, and phospholipid bilayer. Excess extracellular metabolites can force some entry of various substances simply by mass action, such as glucose in the presence of hyperglycemia. Once inside the cytosol, most ions enter freely in equilibrium through the permeable outer mitochondrial membrane. The inner membrane that separates the outer chamber from the inner matrix is a much stronger barrier. It allows almost nothing to enter unless it is metabolically expedient for it to do so. We must understand matrix function since it is the site of ATP formation and, I believe, the core to understanding the abnormality that results in fibromyalgia.

The Krebs cycle produces hydrogen ions (H^+) while generating several tricarboxylic acids. The source of the fuel to be metabolized does not matter to this system. Fats, proteins, and glucose are all equal once they enter this aerobic cycle. The H^+, generated in the tricarboxylic acid cycle is normally maintained only in limited concentrations inside the matrix. The ions are quickly extruded to the outer chamber in a continuous stream, some in the form of NADH, but most via the proton pump. It is imperative that these hydrogen ions (protons) *reenter* the intramembrane space where its electrons drive a complex series of reactions. Electrons that have been released from hydrogen are moved along a chemical production belt in which are embedded NAD, FAD, ubiquinone (Q-10), iron, sulphur-heme compounds, and various cytochromes and are finally introduced to cytochrome c. This sounds complicated, and it is. The gist is that energy is now available to drive a biologic rotor which in turn pushes protons through the ATP synthase enzyme at a site known as F_0. Clockwise spin of the rotor drives hydrogen back into the matrix. In so doing, ATP is formed at a site known as F_1. Counterclockwise spin of that same rotor reverses this process, as ATP is hydrolyzed to provide the required energy to drive hydrogen ions back in the other direction, out of the matrix and into the outer chamber. This rotor system is bidirectional and another wonderful achievement of nature.[39]

As I have stated, I believe phosphate retention begins at a renal level. It is eventually stored to excess within the matrix. Phosphate and hydrogen ions are symported (brought in as a couple) from the outer chamber of the mitochondrion into the matrix. In addition to the effect of excess phosphate, acidifica-

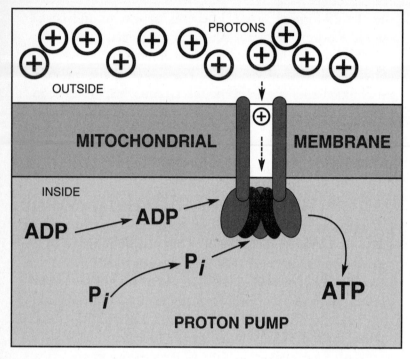

ATP continues to be made as protons move through ATP synthase.

tion of the inner chamber also slows or blocks ATP production. Phosphate can also be countertransported with hydroxyl ions (OH⁻) and gain entry into the matrix without hydrogen ions. However, as matrix acidification proceeds Pi (HPO$_4^=$) increases as well to buffer H⁺ in the form of its equilibrium partner, H$_2$PO$_4^-$.

A paper by Strobel and his associates has utilized ^{31}P magnetic resonance spectroscopy to demonstrate an increase in inorganic phosphate within the contracted muscles of fibromyalgics. They found that as muscle tension develops, pH becomes more alkaline, but, with more prolonged contraction, pH becomes acidic, as in the constantly working tissues of a fibromyalgic. This study is in keeping with the findings of Bengtsson and Henriksson as well as our premise regarding an increase and diprotonation of the mitochondrial Pi, to buffer H$^+$. It is this sequence that leads to the tissue death of ATP and phosphocreatine with consequent dysenergism resulting in system-wide malfunction.[40]

Extracellular chemical, hormonal, or neural impulses stimulate membrane second messengers and trigger calcium sparks from the endoplasmic reticulum. Calcium so released is immediately taken up by contiguous mitochondria, and a far greater amount of calcium is released from the matrix than was taken in initially. This greatly augments the force of the calcium signal and recruits more remote mitochondria to similar action. Calcium drives the cell to the precise level of activity originally requested. Stronger external signals will also open calcium channels and import more of the ions from extracellular sources. The strength of the original, extracellular impulse determines the amount of calcium that will be needed and controls the amplitude of action.

The extrusion of calcium from the mitochondrial matrix is accompanied by potassium in conjunction with hydroxyl ions. As stated in a preceding paragraph, hydroxyl ions are antiported to the outer chamber in exchange for inorganic phosphate (Pi). Symported hydrogen ions can lower pH to the order of plus or minus 6.4. At that level of acidification, ATP production ceases.[41] All of these ionic exchanges are made in the transition permeability pore. This pore cannot remain open and must quickly close. The open state would lead to an excessive loss of ions from critical locations and result in mito-chondrial death (apoptosis).

Muscle fatigue during exercise has been thought to be due to the excess accumulation of lactic acid providing hydrogen ions. However, several authors have challenged this.[42] Their work supports the theory that at least during intense, short-term exercise, the diprotonated, acidic form of inorganic phosphate is the primary companion of fatigue. As stated above, $H_2PO_4^-$ is in equilibrium with inorganic phosphate. During strenuous exercise testing, the diprotonated molecule level rose to an average of more than nine times the resting value. The pH level stabilized at a certain point prior to ending the four-minute exercise, but $H_2PO_4^-$ continued to rise parallel with the increasing level of fatigue. Though pH stabilized, fatigue pro-gressed in parallel with diprotonated phosphate. The con-tracted musculoskeletal lesions palpable in fibromyalgics are low-level, exercising tissues. In their circadian workouts, they accumulate the fatigue molecules (Pi, H^+, $H_2PO_4^-$), which all block ATP generation. Normal exercised tissues eventually rest and are able to purge accumulated, metabolic debris. No such luxury is afforded fibromyalgic tissues. To project this same faulty chemistry onto cells of the intestinal tract, brain, skin, genitourinary system, and so on is only a short step. Work pro-duces metabolites that induce cellular fatigue. The exhaustion expressed by patients is a testimonial to their overworked cells.

We must not forget the constant call to action instigated by the elevated cytosolic calcium ion. Metabolic demands are continuous and fibromyalgic symptoms eventually become so. More hydrogen ion is formed by the overstimulated Krebs cycle in all affected cells, not only musculoskeletal tissues. Gly-colysis is goaded to higher activity in the frenzy to replenish

ATP supplies, and adds to the production of more H^+. This further slows ATP formation since ATP-synthase cannot perform its function unless protons can move bidirectionally. A mitochondrial metabolite must cause the permeability transition pore to close and protect the cell from apoptosis. The mechanism for this is not yet understood.

In summary, we can simplify the above discussion. In fibromyalgia, energy deprivation is initially cyclic, with the brain and other tissues only sporadically affected. Any trigger—either physical or mental—such as trauma, infection, medical or dental interventions, or stress can jump-start the illness. Any call for significant energy expenditure can be the final push to render latent fibromyalgia symptomatic. The brain remembers that carbohydrates are the most effective fuels for rapid production of ATP. Patients often develop carbohydrate craving at this time, but due to metabolic interference, little if any ATP can be formed by yielding to that urge. The increased and repetitive intake of carbohydrates causes equally frequent releases of insulin. This hormone causes an increase in renal reabsorption of inorganic phosphate and promotes its uptake in a variety of cells throughout the body. More phosphate is added to the already overburdened intracellular stores. In genetically susceptible individuals, the hypoglycemia syndrome occurs, with chronic symptoms that overlap those of fibromyalgia. The metabolic mischief created by this combination produces our sickest patients, our "fibroglycemics."

It is imperative that all physicians elicit from patients the symptoms that would point to a defective carbohydrate metabolism. Simply deleting sugars and complex carbohydrates from the diet for a period of two months initiates control of hypoglycemia. The goal of the diet is simple: avoid releasing insulin. Fats release very little insulin. Unless eaten with carbohydrates, proteins release only somewhat more. The rollercoaster rise and fall of glucose is abolished and patients lose all the symptoms related to hypoglycemia.

The low-carbohydrate diet decreases demands for glycolysis, but, through gluconeogenesis provides sufficient glucose for cerebral function and acute needs elsewhere. Certain amino acids and long-chain fatty acids readily enter the matrix and, via the Krebs cycle, provide ample fuel for energy formation. Somewhat less hydrogen ion production results from the dietary change. Because of the diminished insulin pulses, less phosphate is taken up by cells, facilitating the purging by guaifenesin. Thus the diet is helpful for other fibromyalgics, especially those who merely crave carbohydrates but who have not yet developed hypoglycemia.

This chapter is labored with esoteric chemistry, and is complex in its detail. Metabolically oriented journals reveal new information concerning cellular mitochondrial function almost monthly. I have not mentioned newly discovered uncoupling proteins that are currently under heavy scrutiny and are still being defined. They will certainly play a role in fibromyalgia and perhaps they are the proteins that protect cells from apoptosis.

It is certain that I am simplistic in my theoretical design. Changes are so rapid it is likely that I will wish I were able to make many revisions by the time this book goes to press. The biochemistry of living creatures is awesome, as are the perturbations that force patients to our doors. I sincerely hope that this book will help you, physicians, and other professionals better understand what you and they are facing. Fibromyalgics suffer deeply, and desperately need healers to be friends.

Notes

CHAPTER 1

1. Frederick Wolfe, "The Fibromyalgia Problem," *Journal of Rheumatology* 24, no. 7 (1997): 1247–49.

2. W. R. Gowers, "A Lecture on Lumbago: Its Lessons and Analogues," *British Medical Journal* 1 (1904): 117–21.

3. Ibid.

4. F. Wolfe, H. A. Smythe, and M. B. Yunus, "Criteria for the Classification of Fibromyalgia," *The American College of Rheumatology* 33 (1990): 160–72.

5. The Copenhagen Declaration, "Consensus Document on Fibromyalgia," *The Lancet* 240 (September 12, 1992). Incorporated into the ICD on January 1, 1993.

6. F. Wolfe, J. Anderson, and D. Harkness, "The Work and Disability Status of Persons with Fibromyalgia," *Journal of Rheumatology* 24 (1997): 1171–78.

CHAPTER 2

7. Hugh Smythe, "Fibrositis Syndrome: A Historical Perspective," *Journal of Rheumatology* 16, supplement 19 (1989): 2–6.

8. A. Bengtsson and K. G. Henriksson, "The Muscle in Fibromyalgia: A Review of Swedish Studies," *Journal of Rheumatology* 16, supplement 19 (1989): 144–49.

CHAPTER 3

9. Medical Economics, *Physicians' Desk Reference* (Montvale, NJ: Medical Economics, 1999). Entry for Humbid, 1698.

10. C. M. Ramsdell, A. E. Postlewaite, and W. Kelley, "Uricosuric Effect of Glyceryl Guaiacolate," *Journal of Rheumatology* 1, no. 1 (1974): 114–16.

11. Julia Lawless, *The Encyclopedia of Essential Oils* (Lanham, MD: Barnes & Noble, 1992), 106.

12. Medical Economics, *Physicians' Desk Reference for Herbal Medicines* (Montvale, NJ: Medical Economics, 1998).

13. Medical Economics, *Physicians' Desk Reference* (Montvale, NJ: Medical Economics, 1999). Entry for Humbid, 1698.

CHAPTER 4

14. Ilya Raskin, "The Role of Salicylic Acid in Plants," *Annual Review of Plants* 43 (1992): 439–63.

15. P. Morra, W. R. Bartle, and S. E. Walker, "Serum Concentrations of Salicylic Acid Following Topically Applied Salicylate Derivatives," *Ann. Pharmacother.* 9 (September 1996): 935–40.

16. Lillian M. Ingster and Manning Feinleib, paper presented at The American Heart Association—36th Conference on Cardiovascular Disease, Epidemiology, and Prevention, March 1996, San Francisco, CA; P. L. Janssen, P. C. Hollman, and E. Reichman, "Urinary Salicylate Excretion in Subjects Eating a Variety of Diets Shows That Amounts of Bioavailable Salicylates in Food Are Low," *American Journal of Clinical Nutrition* 64 (November 1996): 743–47.

17. A. R. Swain, S. P. Dutton, and A. S. Truswell, "Salicylates in Foods," *Journal of the American Dietetic Association* 85 (August 1998): 950–59.

CHAPTER 5

18. P. Genter and E. Ipp, "Plasma Glucose Thresholds for Counterregulation After an Oral Glucose Load," *Metabolism* 43, no. 1 (January 1994): 98–103.

19. Janette Brand Miller, "International Tables of Glycemic Index," *American Journal of Clinical Nutrition* 62 (1995): 871–90.

20. Robert C. Atkins, *Dr. Atkins' New Diet Revolution* (New York: M. Evans and Co., Inc., 1992); Richard K. Bernstein, *Dr. Bernstein's Diabetes Solution* (New York: Little Brown and Co., 1997).

CHAPTER 7

21. C. C. Solomons, M. H. Melmed, and S. M. Heitler, "Calcium Citrate for Vulvar Vestibulitis: A Case Report," *The Journal of Rep. Med.* 36 (1991): 879–82.

22. J. J. Yount and J. J. Willems, "New Direction in Medical Management of Vulvar Vestibulitis," *Vulvar Pain Newsletter* (Fall 1994): 5–7.

CHAPTER 9

23. Harvey Moldofsky, "Nonrestorative Sleep and Symptoms After a Febrile Illness in Patients with Fibrositis and Chronic Fatigue Syndromes," *Journal of Rheumatology* 16, supplement 19 (1989): 150–53.

CHAPTER 10

24. S. Enestrom, A. Bengtsson, and T. Frodin, "Dermal IgG Deposits and Increase of Mast Cells in Patients with Fibromyalgia: Relevant Findings or Epiphenomena?" *Scandinavian Journal of Rheumatology* 26, no. 4 (1997): 308–13.

CHAPTER 11

25. Origin unknown. The guaiacum entry is from an old book sent to us from a patient in Washington State.

CHAPTER 12

26. Frederick Wolfe, "The Fibromyalgia Problem," *Journal of Rheumatology* 24, no. 7 (1997): 1247–49.

27. Robert Bennett, "Q & A with Robert Bennett, M.D.," *The Fibromyalgia Network Newsletter* (October 1998): 13.

28. Elseviers, Dissertation quoted in "Controversies Surrounding Long-Term Abuse of Analgesics," *The Clinical Courier* 16, no. 14 (August 1997): 4.

29. Don L. Goldenberg, "A Review of the Role of Tricyclic Medications in the Treatment of Fibromyalgia Syndrome," *Journal of Rheumatology* 16, supplement 19 (1989): 137–40.

30. Ibid.

31. Marcia Angell and Jerome P. Kassirer, "Alternative Medicine: The Risks of Untested and Unregulated Remedies," *The New England Journal of Medicine* 339, no. 12 (September 17, 1998): 839–41.

32. Nortin M. Hadler, "Fibromyalgia: La Maladie est Morte. Vive la Malade!" *Journal of Rheumatology* 24, no. 7 (1997): 1250–51.

33. Frederick Wolfe, "Disability and the Distress in Fibromyalgia," *Journal of Musculoskeletal Pain* 1 (1993): 65–87.

CHAPTER 13

34. Devin J. Starlanyl, *The Fibromyalgia Advocate* (Oakland, CA: New Harbinger Publications, 1998), 227.

35. Ibid., 169.

36. Devin J. Starlanyl and Mary Ellen Copeland, *Fibromyalgia and Chronic Myofascial Pain Syndrome: A Survival Manual* (Oakland, CA: New Harbinger Publications, 1996), 161.

TECHNICAL APPENDIX:

37. A. Bengtsson, K. G. Henriksson, and Jorgen Larsson, "Reduced High-Energy Phosphate Levels in the Painful Muscles of Patients with Primary Fibromyalgia," *Arthritis and Rheumatism* 29, no. 7 (July 1986): 817–21.

38. R. M. Bennett, "Beyond Fibromyalgia: Ideas on Etiology and Treatment," *Journal of Rheumatology* 16, supplement 19 (1989): 185–91.

39. X. Kinosita, R. Yasuda, H. NoJi, and M. Yoshida, "F1-ATPase: A Rotary Motor Made of a Single Molecule," *Cell* 93 (April 3, 1998): 21–24.

40. E. S. Strobel, M. Krapf, and M. Suckfüll, "Tissue Oxygen Measurement and ^{31}P Magnetic Resonance Spectroscopy in Patients with Muscle Tension and Fibromyalgia," *Rheumatology International* 16 (1997): 175–80.

41. J. R. Wilson, K. K. McCully, B. B. Mancini, and B. Chance, "Relationship of Muscular Fatigue to pH and Diprotonated P*i* in Humans: A ^{31}P Study," *Journal of Applied Physiology* 64 (1988): 2333-39.

42. J. Eisinger, A. Plantamura, and T. Ayavou, "Glycolysis Abnormalities in Fibromyalgia," *Journal of the American College of Nutrition* 13, no. 2 (1994): 144–48.

Glossary

Acetaminophen (Tylenol®)—an analgesic and antipyretic with effects similar to aspirin, but a weaker anti-inflammatory. "Non-aspirin" pain relievers have this compound as the active ingredient.

Acetic acid—a two-carbon carboxylic acid that gives vinegar its characteristic sour taste. Used in topical preparations to restore acidity of the vagina.

Acid—a donor of hydrogen ions with a positive electrical charge.

Adenosine diphosphate (ADP)—a nucleotide involved in energy metabolism, produced by the hydrolysis of adenosine triphosphate (ATP), and converted back to ATP by the metabolic process, oxidative phosphorylation.

Adenosine triphosphate (ATP)—a biochemical currency of energy that consists of three phosphate molecules and one adenosine molecule. It is vital to our existence, as the body uses it to perform nearly all of its functions.

Adrenaline (epinephrine)—a hormone released by the adrenal glands when the body senses eminent danger. It is sometimes called the "fight or flight hormone." It is designed to increase energy levels in emergencies. When the blood sugar falls in hypoglycemia, the body senses an emergency and releases adrenaline. This release quickly normalizes the blood sugar within one to two minutes.

Alexander Technique—physical therapy that concentrates on correcting body mechanics. It consists of a series of lessons (more than fifteen)—a patient is observed and taught new ways to move to avoid tensed muscles and stress on painful areas.

Allopurinol (Zyloprim®)—a medication for treating gout that blocks the formation of uric acid by inhibiting xanthine oxidase. It does not work for fibromyalgia as do the uricosuric drugs, probenecid and sulfinpyrazone.

Alpha-hydroxyacids—a group of chemically similar acids that are widely used in wrinkle preparations (Glycolic, lactic, malic, citric, and tartaric acids).

Ambien® (zolpiderm tartrate)—a hypnotic sleeping pill for short-term use for insomnia. One of the side-effects of this medication is depression.

Amitripyline (Elavil®)—a commonly used and inexpensive antidepressant that can improve sleep for fibromyalgics. Weight gain, morning drowsiness, dry mouth, and hot flashes are common side effects.

Analgesic drugs—drugs that relieve pain. The two basic types are non-narcotic (containing aspirin or acetaminophen) and narcotics (which are related to morphine). When body tissues are injured they produce prostaglandins. Non-narcotic analgesics (except acetaminophen) block prostaglandin formation. Acetaminophen blocks the pain impulses in the brain. Narcotic analgesics block pain impulses at specific sites called opiate receptors in the brain and spinal cord.

Anergism (absence of energy)—a word we coined for this book. It better describes the true state of fibromyalgia: patient and cellular fatigue. It is not to be confused with "anergy" that defines a poor immune system response.

Angiotensin converting enzyme (kinase II)—an enzyme that catalyzes angiotensin 1 to angiotensin 11.

Antibiotics—a group of drugs effective against bacterial infections. They were originally derived from molds or fungi. Certain antibiotics are effective against different pathogens. Side effects for these drugs vary, but they can all cause the overgrowth of yeast by eliminating the normal microbiota of the gastrointestinal tract.

Antidepressant drugs—a group of medications found to have some value in a limited number of fibromyalgics. Some trigger the release of chemicals in the brain. Others, including the tricylics (see page 361) prolong the active life of chemicals after their release. Common side effects are: dry mouth, dizziness, drowsiness, constipation, and blurry vision.

Antihistamine—drugs used in treating allergies. They counteract the effects of histamines released from mast cells.

Anturane® (sulfinpyrazone)—a medicine used in the treatment of gout. It is uricosuric (causes the kidneys to increase the excretion of uric acid). It was one of our earlier drugs for fibromyalgia.

Apatite—calcium phosphate in a particular chemical structure. It is the main component of dental calculus (tartar).

Apoptosis—programmed cell death.

Aquaphor® lotion—a moisturizing cream that is fragrance-free and preservative-free for severely dry skin. Does not block guaifenesin.

Arnica—herbs of the genus *Arnica*, usually applied topically to reduce pain and inflammation. Blocks guaifenesin.

Aspirin (acetylsalicylic acid)—a synthetic compound used as an antipyretic, analgesic, and anti-inflammatory agent. It interferes with the production of prostaglandins, which are irritants that sensitize pain receptors. Aspirin has effects on many parts of the body, it inhibits platelet aggregation, and has actions in the kidneys as well. Aspirin is known to block uricosuric drugs; in low doses can depress uric acid clearance, and in high doses is uricosuric. It can release thyroid hormone from protein binding and can alter thyroid tests. It can retard the renal elimination of various medications. Overdosage can be fatal.

Atarax® (hydroxyzine HCl.)—an antihistamine that is used primarily for itching since it can cause considerable drowsiness. Has also been used to relieve anxiety.

ATP (adenosine triphosphate)—a biochemical currency of energy that consists of three phosphate molecules and one adenosine molecule. It is vital to our existence, as the body uses it to perform many crucial tasks.

Atypical cystitis—a bladder infection without all the usual characteristics.

Autoimmune diseases—a group of diseases caused when the body produces antibodies that attack its own tissues and cells. More common in women.

Barbiturate—a group of drugs derived from barbituric acid that act as central nervous system depressants. Therefore used as tranquilizers, for seizure control or prevention, and as hypnotics. They have the potential for abuse.

Benadryl® (diphenhydramine)—an inexpensive antihistamine that is also the active ingredient in over-the-counter sleep medications since it causes drowsiness. It is safe for use by children and pregnant women, and is non-habit-forming. (About twenty percent of patients become agitated and cannot use it for sleep.)

Benemid® (probenecid)—a uricosuric sulfa drug used for treating gout. It works by increasing renal excretion of uric acid. It is the first drug we used to treat fibromyalgia.

Betahydroxy acid (BHA)—a group of chemically similar hydroxy acids. In the cosmetic industry and other literature, it is usually synonymous with salicylic acid. It is primarily used for exfoliation (cannot be used with guaifenesin).

Beta-carotene—a substance found in all plants and animals. It is what makes carrots and egg yolks yellow. Its effects are identical to vitamin A. Excesses can cause carotenemia, a yellow, orange, or red pigmentation of the skin.

Bibia—a rare plant sometimes used in expensive cosmetics. Blocks guaifenesin.

Bowen Therapy—a gentle form of body work that uses a light, rolling motion on muscles. It often takes five to ten days for the muscles to respond to this therapy.

Brain cycles—the cognitive symptoms of fibromyalgia—impaired memory and concentration, depression, irritability, nervousness—that come and go in cycles during both the development and the reversal of fibromyalgia.

Brain fog (fibrofog)—a cluster of cognitive symptoms that can last for hours, weeks, or even months. Patients have trouble finding words when speaking, get lost looking for familiar places, transpose numbers, and suffer from impaired short-term memory. It is also described as if a fog exists between a patient and the rest of the world.

Bromelain—an enzyme isolated from papaya and used to aid digestion. Does not block guaifenesin.

Buspar® (buspirone HCl)—An antianxiety drug known to be less sedating than others in its class. It is often prescribed because of its low potential for abuse.

Caffeine—a stimulant drug that occurs in coffee, tea, and cola. Considered the most consumed drug in the United States. It is sometimes added to analgesic medications. It is contraindicated in hypoglycemia because it enhances and prolongs the action of insulin.

Cajeput—white tea tree. Native to Australia and Southeast Asia. Used for arthritis pains and as an anesthetic.

Calcitonin—a hormone secreted primarily by the medullary cells of the thyroid gland. It helps to control the level of calcium in the bloodstream. It deposits calcium and phosphate into bone and also inhibits bone reabsorption, the opposite effects to parathyroid hormone.

Calcium—the most common mineral in the human body. It is essential for all cellular function. It is crucial for muscle contraction, transmission of nerve impulses, blood clotting and, in combination with phosphate, provides the matrix and strength of bone and teeth.

Candida albicans—a yeast (fungus) that can grow in the vagina and rectum. It can grow profusely and cause a thick, cottage-cheese discharge known as candidiasis. Can stem from using antibiotics that excessively kill normal colon or vaginal bacteria. Can also occur in poorly controlled diabetes. Sometimes seen during pregnancy and during menstruation, because of the increased vaginal pH (excessively alkaline).

Capric acid—an acid extracted from a large group of American plants used to make artificial fruit flavors and perfumes. Will not block guaifenesin.

Caprylic triglycerides—a mixture of glycerin with caprylic acid derived from coconut oil. Used in hairspray, lipsticks, and bath oils as an emollient and to help disperse pigment. Will not block guaifenesin.

Carbohydrate intolerance—intended to replace the word hypoglycemia when similar symptoms occur but the blood sugar does not drop below 50 mg/dl. Occurs in forty percent of women fibromyalgics and twenty percent of men. Symptoms are: sugar craving, sweating, hunger tremors, palpitations of the heart, panic attacks, headaches (mainly frontal), dizziness or faintness as well as fatigue, irritability, nervousness, depression, insomnia, poor memory and concentration, and anxieties. These complaints greatly overlap with fibromyalgia.

Carbohydrates—the term includes all sugars and starches. They are composed of carbon, hydrogen, and oxygen and, along with fats, provide the body with its two main sources of energy. Although we usually read about two types of carbohydrates, simple and complex, there are actually three classifications: (a) monosaccharides (glucose, galactose, fructose); (b) disaccharides (sucrose, lactose, maltose); and (c) polysaccharides (starch, cellulose). Ingested carbohydrates raise the blood sugar, causing the pancreas to release insulin. Simple carbohydrates: sugars including table sugar (sucrose), fruit sugar (fructose), honey (maltose), and milk sugar (lactose). Complex carbohydrates: starches such as bread, pasta, rice, potatoes, cereals, peas, and beans.

Cardura® (doxazosin mesylate)—a quinazoline compound used for treating hypertension and bladder neck spasm. Sometimes given prophylactically for headache prevention.

Carisoprodol (Soma®)—a central nervous system depressant that causes muscle relaxation and sometimes helps with the sensory overload symptoms of fibromyalgia. It can cause drowsiness and raise the seizure threshold. It will not block guaifenesin, but soma compound, which contains aspirin, will.

Castor oil—oil from the leaves of the castor plant. It has a powerful laxative action. It is also used in cosmetics, and about fifty percent of lipsticks contain this substance. Will block guaifenesin.

Cataflam® (diclofenac potassium)—a nonsteroidal anti-inflammatory drug with analgesic and antipyretic properties used to treat muscle pain and menstrual cramps.

Cell—the smallest living unit that is able to grow and reproduce. The human body contains billions of cells.

Cell membrane—a double layer of fatty material and proteins that holds the cell together. It also regulates the passage of materials in and out of the cell. Some molecules pass freely, others require special molecular transport systems.

Central nervous system (CNS)—the brain and the spinal cord. It analyzes and responds to sensory information. Analgesics, antidepressants, and sedatives are aimed at slowing or accelerating the function of this system.

Centrax® (prazepam)—a benzodiazepine, antianxiety drug that is also used to treat insomnia and muscle spasm. Side effects include drowsiness, dizziness, and confusion. If used for two weeks or more, this class of drugs must be discontinued slowly to avoid withdrawal symptoms.

Cetyl alcohol—an emollient used in many cosmetics and hair products. Also used as a laxative. Derived from spermaceti of the sperm whale.

Chlamydia—a gram-negative bacteria that can cause a variety of diseases in humans (and animals) including trachoma, inclusion conjunctivitis (or inclusion blennorrhea) as well as "nonspecific" urethritis and prostatitis.

Choline salicylate (Arthropan®)—a salicylate compound sometimes used for the pain of arthritis. It will block guaifenesin.

Chronic—something that has persisted for a long time.

Chronic candidiasis—a chronic infection attributed to the overgrowth of candida albicans.

Chronic fatigue syndrome (CFIDS, chronic fatigue immune dysfunction syndrome, or "yuppie flu")—a complex of symptoms, the dominant one being severe fatigue defined as more than six months' duration. This fatigue is not caused by exertion and is not relieved by rest. CFIDS patients commonly suffer headaches, sore throats, muscle and joint pain, and weakness. Most doctors now consider CFIDS and FMS to be the same disorder, with patients at opposite ends of a spectrum of symptoms.

Clotrimazole—a broad-spectrum antifungal agent, applied topically to the skin in the treatment of candidiasis and various forms of tinea; administered intravaginally for treatment of vulvovaginal candidiasis.

Cocamidopropyl—a chemical extracted from the kernels of the coconut.

Codeine—a narcotic derived from opium or morphine and used as a cough suppressant, analgesic, and hypnotic.

Colonoscopy—a medical procedure that examines the colon. An *endoscope* (colonoscope) is inserted rectally and passed upward. The instrument is gradually withdrawn as the walls of the colon are inspected. It is usually done in a doctor's office or hospital "GI lab" with the patient mildly sedated.

Connective tissue—the material that holds structures of the body together; includes tendons, cartilage, and the nonmuscular structures of arteries and veins.

Constipation—difficult or infrequent elimination of hard, dry stools. A common symptom of fibromyalgia.

Corticosteroid drugs—drugs similar to the natural corticosteroid hormones produced by the adrenal gland. Used to treat inflammatory bowel disease, asthma, rheumatoid arthritis, adrenal insufficiency, and some skin problems. They may be injected into painful muscles or joints to relieve pain. They suppress the immune system, can cause the loss of bone density, and suppress the action of the adrenal gland. They must be discontinued slowly under a doctor's supervision.

Cortisol—the normal corticosteroid hormone released by the adrenal glands that contributes to the metabolism of nutrients; helps to control the retention of salt and water while eliminating potassium.

Cortisone—a natural hormone from the adrenal gland that is produced synthetically. It exerts its pharmaceutical effects by conversion to cortisol. It is used in replacement therapy for adrenal insufficiency and as an anti-inflammatory and immunosuppressant in a wide variety of disorders; administered orally and intramuscularly.

Capsaicin—a location compound used for pain, itching, and neuropathies. It apparently works by depleting Substance P and other peptide pain mediators. It is made from chili peppers and will block guaifenesin.

Craniosacral therapy (craniosacral release, CSR)—a gentle type of body work based on correcting blocks in the craniosacral system (brain, spinal cord, cerebrospinal fluid, the cranial bones, and the sacrum).

Cycling—describes the alternating between better and worse days. Intensification of cycling (or cycles) is the hallmark of fibromyalgia reversal with guaifenesin. Commonly used by patients to describe a period of bad days.

Cyclobenzaprine (Flexeril®)—a tricyclic medication shown to have some benefits in fibromyalgia. Used to relax muscle spasms, and induce Stage 4 sleep. The primary side effects are drowziness, morning somnolence, and dry mouth.

Cyclomethicone—one of many silicone oils used in cosmetics. It leaves the skin silky and is a water-binding agent. It will not block guaifenesin.

Cystitis—inflammation of the urinary bladder. Common symptoms are urinary frequency and pain on bladder filling and at the end of urination. Bacterial cystitis is a bacterial infection of the bladder. Interstitial cystitis is a chronic disorder of the bladder occurring predominantly in women and notoriously difficult to detect.

Cystogram—a radiograph of the bladder.

Cystoscope—a fiber-optic scope used in the urinary tract. It is inserted through the urethra up into the bladder to permit visualization of the lining structures and orifices.

Cystoscopy—the procedure using a cystoscope for the above purposes. Usually done under mild sedation and with a local anesthetic.

Cytokines—powerful chemical substances released by cells when in contact with an antigen. They act as intercellular mediators such as in the generation of immune responses.

Cytoplasm—fluid material inside a cell, as distinct from structures such as the nucleus and organelles.

Darvocet-N® (propoxyphene napsylate and acetaminophen)—a centrally acting narcotic analgesic related to methadone. Dizziness, sedation, and nausea are the primary side effects. It is considered potentially addictive.

Darvon® (propoxyphene hydrochloride)—a centrally acting narcotic analgesic related to methadone. Dizziness, sedation, and nausea are the primary side effects. Is considered potentially addictive.

Darvon Compound®—same as above, except that it contains aspirin. Will block guaifenesin.

Daypro® (oxaprozin)—a nonsteroidal anti-inflammatory drug with some analgesic effects. Used for muscle pain.

Dental calculus (tartar)—hard, crust-like deposit on the roots and crowns of teeth. Formed from saliva as mineral salt deposits of calcium and phosphate to encrust plaque, debris, and dead bacteria.

Dental plaque—a soft, thin film of food debris, mucin, and dead epithelial cells deposited on the teeth, providing a medium for bacterial growth. The main inorganic components are calcium and phosphate. It provides the base for the development of dental calculus.

Dermatographia—a skin condition where one can use a fingernail or blunt instrument and literally write on the patient's skin. This causes surface redness from the swelling of the dermal capillaries that renders the written inscriptions visible.

Dermis—the sensitive connective tissue layer of the skin located deep to the epidermis (outer layer of the skin). It contains nerve endings, sweat and sebaceous glands, and blood and lymph vessels.

Desyrel® (trazodone)—an antidepressant commonly used especially for those with sleep problems. Common side effects are somnolence, dizziness, and dry mouth.

Dextromethorphan (DM)—an antitussive agent that has no addictive or analgesic effect. It is used in cough medicines to raise the cough threshold.

Dextroretroverted uterus—a tilted ("tipped") uterus that bends to the right and backward.

Dextrose—a monosaccharide known as glucose in biochemistry. Common constituent of foods and intravenous feedings.

DHEA (dehydroepiandrosterone)—the most abundant hormone produced by the adrenal glands; levels fall with age. It is a pro-hormone used for the formation of estrogen and testosterone.

Diabetes—a syndrome due to impaired carbohydrate metabolism because of insufficient secretion of insulin or by the insulin resistance of target tissues, mainly muscle and fat cells. It occurs in two major forms: insulin-dependent diabetes mellitus (Type I) and non-insulin-dependent diabetes mellitus (Type II), which differ in etiology, pathology, genetics, age of onset, and treatment. Type I diabetes mellitus (also called growth-onset or juvenile-onset diabetes, insulin-dependent diabetes, or IDDM) is characterized by abrupt onset of symptoms—the usual age of onset is twelve years—but can occur at any age. The disorder is due to lack of insulin production by the beta cells of the pancreatic islets. This form of diabetes is treated with insulin, and cannot be controlled by dietary restriction alone. Type II diabetes mellitus (adult-onset, non-insulin-dependent diabetes, or NIDDM) has a gradual onset. Dietary (carbohydrate) restriction and weight loss can control this form of diabetes in the earlier stages. The average age of onset is fifty to sixty years. Genetic tendencies and obesity are the two risk factors for this type of diabetes. Subclinical diabetes is impaired glucose tolerance without symptoms. Gestational diabetes is a carbohydrate intolerance with onset during pregnancy. Women with this form of diabetes are at increased risk for developing Type II diabetes.

Diflucan® (fluconazole)—an antifungal medication often prescribed for systemic candidiasis. A single dose is also used to treat a vaginal yeast infection. It penetrates all of the body tissues. Long-term use of this medication requires monitoring of liver function.

Dimethicone—a silicone oil used in hair products and cosmetics. Derived from silica, and can be used with guaifenesin.

Diphenhydramine (Benadryl®)—an inexpensive antihistamine that is also the active ingredient in over-the-counter sleep medications. It is safe for use by children and pregnant women, and is non-habit-forming. (About twenty percent of patients become agitated and cannot use it for sleep.)

Disaccharide—a carbohydrate consisting of two of the same or different sugar molecules. Sucrose, lactose, and maltose are disaccharides.

Diverticulitis—inflammation or infection of small protrusions from the colon known as diverticula. These are similar to the tip of a balloon that has not been completely inflated. Usually develops in the lower (sigmoid) colon. Antibiotics are normally prescribed to prevent perforation and peritonitis.

Dolorimeter—a spring-loaded device designed to provide a measurement for the point at which a patient flinches or expresses pain.

Double-blind study—a medical study used to test the efficacy of a treatment. One half of the patients are treated, and the other half receive a placebo, or nonmedication. Neither the patient nor the person conducting the study knows who is receiving the drug and who is not. Thus the name "double-blind."

Doxepin (Sinequan®)—an antidepressant drug with a strong sedating effect. Used for depression and insomnia. Side effects include dry mouth, blurred vision, and drowsiness. Maximum effects require two to six weeks.

Doxycycline—a tetracycline antibiotic drug commonly used for prostatitis, urethritis, and pelvic inflammatory diseases. The absorption of this drug, unlike the other tetracyclines, is not affected if taken with food.

Drowsiness—an altered state between full wakefulness and sleep.

Drug—a chemical substance that alters the function of one or more body organs or changes the course and symptoms of a disease. The term includes over-the-counter (nonprescription), prescription, and illicit drugs. Some foods and drinks contain substances considered drugs, such as caffeine. A drug can have three designations, a chemical, a generic, and a specific brand name. Originally all drugs were natural substances from plants, animals, or minerals. Today most drugs are produced in laboratories, ensuring a predictable potency and purity.

Drug addiction—the metabolic demand by the brain that is enslaved to a substance to such an extent that withdrawal causes intense symptoms and a pathologic drive to surmount all obstacles to its procurement.

Drug dependence—a lesser form of addiction. It is a strong need to continue taking a drug either to prevent withdrawal effects or to obtain a desired effect. Medically speaking, cigarette smoking is considered a drug dependency. There are two kinds of drug dependence—mental and physical.

Drug tolerance—the situation where an increasingly higher amount of a drug is needed to produce the same effects previously obtained at a lower dosage. It is usually caused by the liver's becoming more efficient at breaking down the drug, or to the body's decreasing sensitivity to the substance.

Dysenergism syndrome (defective energy)—a name coined for this book, which along with anergism, is a more descriptive name for the disease currently called "fibromyalgia." Both of these names describe the patients' symptoms and the actual, biochemical fatigue within their cells.

Dysmenorrhea—pain during or just before a menstrual period. Includes cramps, backache, nausea, and vomiting.

Dyspareunia—painful sexual intercourse.

Dyspepsia—indigestion.

Dysphagia—difficulty swallowing.

Dysuria—discomfort during urination expressed as pain or burning; also difficulty in passing urine.

Eczema—an inflammation of the skin that produces itchy, scaly patches with tiny blisters, cracking, and weeping areas. There are many types of eczema, including neuro or seborrheic dermatitis.

Edema—an abnormal accumulation of serum-like fluid in the body tissues.

Effexor® (venlafaxine HCl)—an antidepressant that inhibits serotonin and norepinephrine reuptake. May suppress pain perception. This medication must be tapered off gradually when discontinued. Side effects include hair loss, dry mouth, and drowsiness.

Elavil® (amitriptyline)—a commonly used and inexpensive antidepressant that can improve sleep and suppress pain perception. Weight gain and morning drowsiness are two common side effects.

ELISA test (enzyme-linked immunosorbent assay)—a laboratory test used in the diagnosis of various diseases.

Elmiron® (pentosan polysulfate sodium)—a drug used to treat interstitial cystitis by binding to the lining of the bladder. Side effects are rare and include headache, abdominal pain, and diarrhea.

Empirin® (aspirin)—a 325 mg aspirin and caffeine tablet. Will block guaifenesin.

Endocrine system—made up of glands that produce hormones (chemicals necessary for many bodily functions) which regulate or stimulate metabolism, growth, sexual development, and function; powerful components necessary to maintain the body in a state of balance (known as homeostasis).

Endocrinology—a medical specialty that focuses on the study of the glands that produce hormones, the hormones themselves, and their effects on the body.

Endoplasmic reticulum—a complex organelle within cells responsible for the production of various proteins such as enzymes. It stores calcium that can be released on command, the final signal that drives a cell to perform its assigned functions.

Endorphins—hormones released by the body in response to acute pain; the body's own natural painkillers. Endorphins are natural opioids that block pain receptors. They are one reason why we do not feel acute pain immediately after an injury.

Endoscopy—a procedure done with a fiber-optic instrument enabling direct visual examination. A long, narrow tube is inserted through the mouth into the esophagus, stomach, and duodenum, the first part of the small intestine. A term also used for a similar procedure in any other part of the body.

Energy—the capacity to effect a physical change. The most important forms of energy in the human body are chemical and thermal. It is derived from foods, especially carbohydrates and fats (less by proteins), and is stored in a chemical form as ATP.

Enzymes—proteins that function as biochemical catalysts to regulate the rate and extent of chemical reactions in the body. They are conjugates that derive some of their characteristics from chemical bonding with certain carbohydrates and metals such as calcium, magnesium, zinc, etc.

Epinephrine—a hormone, also known as adrenaline, released by the adrenal glands when the body senses eminent internal or external danger. It is sometimes called the "fight-or-flight hormone." It is designed to increase energy levels in emergencies, for example in hypoglycemia. It is intricately involved in metabolism and day to day nutritional control.

Epstein-Barr virus (EB virus)—a virus that causes infectious mononucleosis once thought to be the cause of chronic fatigue syndrome.

Ergot—a product extracted from a fungus grown on rye and other grains. Ergotamine, used to treat migraine headaches, is produced from this substance. It constricts dilated blood vessels and is used in the very early stages of a migraine attack.

Essential oils (volatile oils)—oily liquids obtained from plants through a variety of processes. They are potent to the extent that a teaspoon can cause illness, and less than an ounce can kill an adult. They block guaifenesin.

Estradiol—the body's natural and most potent estrogen, the female sex hormone. It is synthesized and used to treat the symptoms of menopause, reduce the risk of osteoporosis, and to prevent arteriosclerosis. It is also prescribed in a cream form to treat vaginal dryness and vulvar pain.

Estrogens—a group of hormones produced mainly in the ovaries, but produced in small amounts in both men and women by the adrenal glands and fat cells. These hormones control female sexual development and the functioning of the reproductive system.

Etodolac (Lodine®)—a nonsteroidal anti-inflammatory drug with some analgesic and antipyretic effects. Side effects include stomach pain and diarrhea, and the risk of GI bleeding.

Fascia—fibrous connective tissue that surrounds many of the structures of the body.

Fatty acids—acids containing carbon, hydrogen, and oxygen; the main constituents of fats. Over forty kinds are found in nature. Two are known as the essential fatty acids (linoleic and linolenic acids), meaning that they cannot be made by the body and must be ingested.

Feldenkrais Method—a movement therapy where body movements are integrated to lessen effort and pain.

Ferrous sulfate—an iron compound often given for anemia.

Fibrocystic breast disease—single or multiple benign tumors or cysts in the breast. It is considered unrelated to fibromyalgia, though observations continue in this regard.

Fibroflux—a term coined by Dr. Devin Starlanyl, M.D., to describe the fluctuating emotions due to hormonal changes in fibromyalgics.

Fibrofog—a term used to describe the cognitive impairments of fibromyalgia.

Fibrofrustration—an intense frustration caused by dealing with fibrofog, fibroflux, and physical pain and incapacity. A term coined for this book.

Fibroglycemia—a name coined for this book to describe patients who suffer from both fibromyalgia and carbohydrate intolerance.

Fibrogut—a descriptive name coined for this book to describe the irritable bowel syndrome and other gastrointestinal symptoms of fibromyalgia.

Fibromyalgia—a term that literally means pain in the muscles and fibers. It poorly describes the illness and we suggest replacing it with either dysenergism or anergism.

Fiorinal® (butalbital, aspirin, and caffeine), Fioricet® (butalbital, acetaminophen, and caffeine)—a medication that combines analgesics (aspirin or acetaminophen) with a barbituate (butalbital) to achieve muscle relaxation and reduce anxiety, and with caffeine to counteract drowsiness. Prescribed primarily for "tension headaches." Can cause rebound headaches and side effects such as drowsiness, dizziness, and stomach upset. Patients may develop a tolerance and physical dependence to this medication.

Flagyl® (metronidazole)—a medication used for treatment of trichomoniasis (a one-celled organism), various intestinal parasites, and bacteria. It has many side effects including nausea, headaches, and diarrhea.

Flare—an intensification of symptoms, sometimes called a "fibro-flare or cycle."

Flatulence—intestinal gas.

Flexeril® (cyclobenzaprine)—a tricyclic medication that relaxes and eases muscle twitching and spasms. It induces drowsiness, which may help with sleep but can cause stomach upset, daytime somnolence, and a dry mouth.

Flexin®—a muscle relaxant and potently uricosuric drug highly effective for fibromyalgia. It was withdrawn from the market due to serious side effects.

Fluconazole (Diflucan®)—an antifungal medication often prescribed for systemic candidiasis. A single dose is sufficient to treat a vaginal yeast infection. It penetrates all of the body tissues. Prolonged use of this medication requires monitoring of liver function.

FMS (fibromyalgia syndrome)—a common acronym for fibromyalgia.

Fructose (fruit sugar)—the naturally occurring sugar in fruit that is assigned a reading of 50 on the glycemic index of foods.

Galactose—a sugar derived from lactose in milk; assigned a reading of 43 on the glycemic index of foods.

Gamma globulin—a substance prepared from human blood that contains antibodies against many common infections.

Gastritis—inflammation of the mucous membranes that line the stomach. It can be caused by a drug such as aspirin, anti-inflammatories, alcohol, or by an infection. It can also be triggered by severe physical or mental stress.

Gastroesophageal reflux—a condition caused by acid regurgitation from the stomach back into the esophagus. It can cause esophageal spasms and chest pain that closely mimics cardiac pain.

Generic drug—a medicinal drug marketed under its chemical name. When the patent expires on a drug, companies other than the original manufacturer are at liberty to produce and market a cheaper substitute.

Genome—the complete genetic map of an organism. In a human being a haploid set (from one parent only) contains abut three billion base pairs of DNA and approximately 100,000 genes.

Glucagon—a hormone secreted by the pancreas that stimulates the breakdown of glycogen (the storage form of carbohydrate in the liver and muscles) into glucose. It helps regulate blood glucose levels and opposes the action of insulin.

Glucose—the body's chief source of rapid energy. It can be derived from ingested carbohydrates or produced in cells from fats and proteins (gluconeogenesis). It is found naturally in such foods as grapes and corn. It is 100 on the glycemic index, and on this particular scale is the basis of comparison for all other foods.

Glucose tolerance test—tests the body's ability to absorb and clear glucose from the blood. A specific amount of glucose is ingested, and blood samples are drawn at designated times and tested for glucose (blood sugar) levels. The ability to clear glucose from the blood within specified times determines a patient's "glucose tolerance."

Glycemic index of foods—ranks foods by how they affect blood sugar levels in comparison with pure glucose. (Initially devised with glucose as 100, it is now more common in America to see white bread set at the 100 point. In this book, we use the original scale with glucose as 100. To use white bread as the baseline, multiply the glucose scale by 0.7.)

Glycerides—naturally occurring fats or those made synthetically from glycerin. Used as emollients in cosmetics. Will not block guaifenesin.

Glycerin—a by-product from soap manufacture; used in many products as a solvent, humectant, and emollient. Will not block guaifenesin.

Glycerol—another name for glycerin (see above).

Glycogen—the major storage form of glucose within muscles and liver. It is readily broken down to meet energy needs.

Gout—a predominantly male disease caused by the excess production or renal retention of uric acid (urate). Manifested by recurrent, painful, acute inflammatory arthritis of the lower extremities as well as kidney stones. It is diagnosed by a blood test showing an elevated serum uric acid.

Growing pains—vague aches and pains that occur usually in the legs and at night in children between six and twelve years of age.

Growth hormone (GH, somatotropin)—a hormone secreted by the anterior pituitary. It affects protein, carbohydrate, and lipid metabolism, and controls the rate of skeletal and visceral growth. One of the hormones sometimes found in the low normal range in fibromyalgics.

Guaiacolate—a purified form of tree bark extract that was used in some cough preparations. It was later synthesized and named guaifenesin.

Guaiacum—the natural form of guaifenesin extracted from a tree bark; used in cough medicines and in treating growing pains in children. First mentioned in 1530 A.D. to treat rheumatism.

Guaifenesin (glyceryl guaiacolate)—a medication available in both over-the-counter (200 mg) and prescription strengths (600, 1200 mg). Used to loosen and liquefy mucus. Guaifenesin has no serious side effects. The many symptoms that occur with its use are due to clearing of fibromyalgic debris from the multiple sites of disease involvement. It is minimally uricosuric, and produces an increase in urinary 5-hydroxyindoleacetic acid, the excreted form of serotonin.

Habituation—formation of a habit, used to describe a drug dependence.

Half-life—the time required for the body to eliminate enough of a drug so that only half of the original amount remains in the blood stream. Used to measure how long drugs remain in the body and to gauge the duration of their action.

Hematuria—blood in the urine.

Herb—a plant with a fleshy stem often used in seasoning or medicinally. Herbs concentrated in medications will block guaifenesin because of their salicylate content. The small amounts used in cooking pose no problem.

Hismanal® (astemizole succinate)—a prescription antihistamine used to treat allergies. Unlike most antihistamines, it rarely causes drowsiness.

Histamine—a chemical produced mainly in mast cells; released from exposure to certain irritants such as in allergic reactions. It is one cause of inflammation. It stimulates stomach acid production, narrows the airways in the lungs, causes skin rashes such as hives and many other systemic effects.

Hives (urticaria)—a skin condition characterized by intensely itching welts. Hives are considered an allergic reaction to an internal or external agent. Sometimes attributed to nervousness. Common in fibromyalgia, they are caused by the release of histamines in the tissues under the skin.

Homeopathy—a system of medical treatment based on the use of small quantities of a substance that in larger doses produces symptoms similar to the disease being treated.

Hormones—chemicals necessary to regulate the body's functions. They regulate or stimulate metabolism, growth, sexual development, and function, and maintain the body in a state of balance (known as homeostasis).

Hyaluronic acid—a natural protein found in the fluids around joints. Used in cosmetics.

Hydrocodone—a semisynthetic narcotic derivative of codeine having sedative and analgesic effects more powerful than those of codeine.

Hydrocortisone—a corticosteroid drug used to treat inflammatory disorders and allergies. It is chemically identical to cortisol. Produced by the adrenal glands. In excess or with prolonged use, it has many serious side effects such as thinning skin, diabetes, hypertension, atherosclerosis, muscle atrophy, glaucoma, ulcers, and osteoporosis.

Hydrogenated soy glyceride—a liquid fat extracted from soybean to which hydrogen has been added under high pressure.

Hydrogenation—a process where hydrogen gas is added under high pressure to liquid oils (fats). It is used in the cosmetic industry to change liquid oils to semisolid fats at room temperature. Reduces spoilage and degradation.

Hyperuricemia—high levels of serum uric acid characteristic of gout.

Hypoglycemia—from the Greek "*hypo*" meaning low, sugar (*glyc*) in the blood (*emia*). The accepted medical criterion for this condition is a blood sugar reading falling below 50 mg/dl.

Ibuprofen—a nonsteroidal anti-inflammatory drug marketed in both over-the-counter (Advil®) and prescription (Motrin®) strengths. Side effects include abdominal pain, diarrhea, nausea, heartburn, and dizziness.

Imipramine (Tofranil®)—the original tricyclic antidepressant. Side effects include drowsiness, dizziness, fatigue, headaches, and dry mouth.

Imitrex® (sumatriptan)—a prescription medication used for migraines; administered orally, by injection, or by nasal spray. It cannot be used to prevent migraines, but is for the relief of symptoms. It acts upon specific serotonin receptors in the brain.

Immune system—guards against foreign or disease-producing substances such as bacteria and viruses. The major components of the system are the white blood cells and the antibodies they produce.

Immunoglobulin G—one of the five classes of antibodies that serves many functions. It is often the mediator of autoimmune reactions that result in rashes and more serious symptoms.

Inderal (propranolol HCl)—originally designed as a blood pressure medication, sometimes used to slow the heart rate, block the effects of epinephrine, or to prevent migraines. The primary side effects are lowered blood pressure, slowed heart rate, depression, and decreased energy.

Inflammation—swelling, redness, heat, and pain in tissues due to an injury or infection. It is caused by the release of products from mast cells. Histamines increase the blood flow to the area, causing the redness and heat. It is usually accompanied by the accumulation of white blood cells.

Ingestion—taking a substance into the body through the mouth.

Inguinal ligaments—double, parallel cords that are present on each side of the groin and run from the pelvic bone in front of the hip to the pubic bone. The abdominal muscles actually form the ligament as they curl around each other and make the rope-like structure that attaches and secures them.

Inhibitors—agents that block the actions of another.

Inorganic phosphate (orthophosphate)—an anion or salt of orthophosphoric acid or of any of its esters; it is the major intracellular anion. Abbreviated Pi. The chemical formula is $HPO_4 = Pi$.

Insulin—the only hormone that can direct excess calories (energy) into storage. It is released promptly when carbohydrates are eaten, and begins working even before the meal is completed. Insulin is an insurance hormone that saves surplus calories from each meal for future energy needs.

Interstitial cystitis—a bladder disease defined by the absence of positive tests for other bladder conditions, manifested by bladder and pelvic pain, and the constant urge to urinate that produces only a small amount of urine. It is more prevalent in females than males.

Intracellular—inside the cell.

Ion—an atom or a molecule that has acquired an electric charge by gaining or losing one or more electrons.

Irritable bowel syndrome—a condition that is manifested by excess gas, abdominal pain, bloating, constipation alternating with diarrhea, and sometimes, nausea, hyperacidity, and mucus in the stool. Very common in fibromyalgics.

Isomethephene mucate (Midrin®)—a compound used to treat headache pain, both vascular and tension. Side effects are dizziness and skin rash.

Jojoba—a shrub native to the southwest United States and northern Mexico with leaves and edible fruit that contain an oil used in cosmetics and moisturizing creams. Blocks guaifenesin.

Ketosis—a condition that results from the body burning fats for fuel instead of glucose.

Klonopin® (klonazepam)—an antianxiety medication, also an anticonvulsive and antispasmodic. It is used to help with sleep and to control the restless leg syndrome. Side effects include fatigue and dizziness.

Lac-Hydrin® (ammonium lactate)—a 12% alpha-hydroxy lotion or cream used to treat severely dry skin or ichthyosis (scaly skin). It requires a prescription, but there is an over-the-counter version known as Lac-Hydrin Five.

Lactose (milk sugar)—a sugar formed by combining glucose and galactose. Rated 48 on the glycemic index of foods, it is permitted on the liberal diet for hypoglycemia. Lactose intolerance is caused by the lack of the enzyme lactase. It is also used as a base in eye lotions, as a filler in pharmaceuticals, and in cosmetics. Will not block guaifenesin.

Lanolin—an oil obtained from sheep's wool used as an emollient.

Librax®—an antispasmodic and tranquilizer used to relieve the symptoms of the irritable bowel syndrome. Side effects include drowsiness, confusion, water retention, nausea, and constipation. It should be discontinued gradually since withdrawal symptoms can occur.

Ligaments—fibrous tissues that connect or tie together bones or cartilage. They are pliant, flexible, and strong.

Lipids—a group of fats that include triglycerides (the principal component of body fat), cholesterol, and high-density lipoprotein (the "good cholesterol").

Liver function tests—blood tests that detect abnormalities in the liver such as inflammation or malfunction. The most common tests are the ALT (SGPT) and AST (SGOT).

Lodine® (etodolac)—a nonsteroidal anti-inflammatory drug with some analgesic and antipyretic effects. Side effects are similar for this entire class of drugs and include stomach upset (gastritis), dizziness, depression, constipation, or diarrhea. The most serious side effect is the risk of gastrointestinal bleeding.

Lorcet® (hydrocodone bitartrate and acetaminophen)—a more potent version of Vicodin. It has a high potential for abuse; side effects are fatigue, dizziness, mental confusion, nausea, and somnolence. May cause liver damage.

Lumbago—lower back pain.

Lumbar area—the lower portion of the back from the back of the rib cage to the sacrum.

Lupus—a group of diseases but usually used to designate systemic lupus erythematosus. Affects the skin and joints but can also attack the kidneys, liver, and brain. Some of the symptoms of lupus may be similar to fibromyalgia, but it can usually be distinguished by blood tests.

Magnesium salicylate (Magam®)—a drug used to treat arthritis pain, and inflammation. It will block guaifenesin.

Maltose (malt sugar)—a sugar formed during the digestion of some starches rated 110 on the glycemic index of food.

Mapping—our term for the manual examination of a patient. It is used to find the lesions, the swollen tissues of fibromyalgia (spastic muscles, tendons, ligaments, and even joints). The findings are drawn on a printed caricature of the body. The size, shape, and location of each abnormality is depicted and shaded according to the degree of hardness. The system is used as a baseline for future, similar drawings to monitor the progress of treatment.

Mast cells—cells found in many tissues but most prevalently in the innermost layer of the skin. They are known to release histamine, heparin (an anticoagulant), interleukins, and as many as thirty other proteins (cytokines). They are found in the skin of fibromyalgics, bladder of patients with interstitial cystitis, and in the bronchial tree of asthmatics.

MCS—see multiple chemical sensitivities.

Melatonin—a hormone from the pineal gland whose full effects are unknown but has been called the sleep hormone. It also affects mood, puberty, and ovarian cycles. It is available without prescription to induce sleep and to counter jet lag. It is commonly administered sublingually for a more rapid action. The primary side effect is depression.

Metabolism—a term for the chemical processes that take place in the body.

Methadone—a synthetic narcotic painkiller primarily used to treat withdrawal symptoms from addiction to other narcotics. It causes milder symptoms though it is chemically related. Side effects include nausea, dizziness, constipation, and dry mouth.

Methyl salicylate (oil of wintergreen)—used as a local anesthetic and disinfectant. Derived from sweet birch, cassie, and wintergreen leaves. Readily absorbed through the skin and toxic when ingested. Lethal dose is 10 cc for children, 30 cc in adults. Will block guaifenesin.

Midrin® (isometheptene mucate, dichloralphenazone and acetaminophen)—a compound used to treat both vascular and tension headaches. The main side effects are dizziness and skin rash.

Migraine—a severe headache that may be accompanied by visual disturbances, nausea, and vomiting. Three times more common in women than in men.

Minerals—inorganic materials found in the earth's crust. Will not block guaifenesin.

Mitochondria—the power stations inside almost all cells in the body. They are complex energy-producing factories that convert about eighty percent of our ingested food into the currency of energy, or ATP. Their disturbed metabolism is our candidate as the cause of the ravages of fibromyalgia.

Molecule—group of atoms held together by chemical forces.

Monosaccharides—a simple sugar; a carbohydrate consisting of a single molecule. Glucose, galactose, and fructose are monosaccharides.

MPS—see myofascial pain syndrome.

Mucolytic agent—a substance that liquefies mucus. Helps loosen and clear mucus from the respiratory passages. Also used in higher dosages to liquefy the normal cervical plug and thereby facilitate conception.

Mucus—the slimy, slippery discharge from certain membranes such as the nose, bronchial tubes, vaginal, or rectal lining. Used by the body as a protective lubricant.

Multiple chemical sensitivities—conditions that arise from exposure to environmental chemicals, various pollutants such as smog, industrial chemicals, pesticides, food additives, preservatives, perfumes, etc.

Muscle—tissue composed of fibers capable of movement by coordinated contraction and relaxation.

Muscle-relaxant drugs (carisoprodol, diazepam, methocarbamol, baclofen, etc.)—used to relieve muscle spasms; work by partially blocking nerve signals from the brain and spinal cord that stimulate contraction. Side effects include weakness, drowsiness, and slowing of mental processes.

Mycostatin® (nystatin)—an antifungal antibiotic drug administered orally and topically.

Myofascial pain syndrome (MPS)—a condition manifested by multiple trigger points in all parts of the body that have been present for at least six months. This group of symptoms comes from problems with the fascia, a band of fibrous tissue that lies deep under the skin and supports muscles and other body organs.

Myofascial therapy—physical therapy designed to relieve muscle and tissue spasms; begins with passive stretching and craniosacral and myofascial release.

Naproxen (sodium) (Naprosyn®, Anaprox®, Aleve®)—a nonsteroidal, anti-inflammatory drug marketed in both prescription and over-the-counter strengths. Used for treating muscle pain, gout, inflammation, menstrual cramps, etc. Side effects are the same as the entire class of drug, including abnormal liver function, headaches, depression, and insomnia.

Narcotics—drugs derived from opium or opium-like compounds with potent analgesic effects. They alter mood and behavior, and induce sedation. They have a high potential for tolerance and addiction.

Nervous system (CNS, central nervous system)—cells, tissues, and organs that regulate bodily responses to internal and external stimuli. The brain, spinal cord, nerves, and ganglia make up the system.

Neuralgia—repeated bolts of pain that radiate along the course of one or more nerves.

Neurodermatitis—an extremely variable type of eczema that is attributed to many causes.

Neurontin® (gabapentin)—an anticonvulsive drug. The mechanism by which this drug works is unknown. Side effects include somnolence, dizziness, and fatigue.

Neuropeptide Y—a hormone released from the hypothalamus at the base of the brain. It is the hormone that induces hunger.

Neurotransmitters—molecules released from nerve cells that carry chemical messages across the minute distance between two nerve cells and deliver them by binding to a receptor on the second nerve.

Nonsteroidal anti-inflammatory drugs (NSAIDs)—nonsalicylate drugs that reduce fever, pain, and inflammation by blocking the formation of prostaglandins. They are available both over the counter (ibuprofen, naproxen) and by prescription (etodolac, oxaprozin, etc.). They must be used with caution because they can cause chemical hepatitis and gastrointestinal bleeding. New evidence suggests they may inhibit energy production. They are of questionable value in fibromyalgia, where no inflammation is present, though they afford some pain relief.

Norepinephrine—a neurotransmitter with some effects similar to epinephrine. It innervates different tissues. One of the group known as catecholamines.

Norepinephrine uptake inhibitors—drugs that prolong the effects of norepinephrine by delaying its uptake and destruction by tissues.

NSAIDs—see nonsteroidal anti-inflammatory drugs.

Nystatin (Mycostatin®)—antifungal antibiotic drug administered orally and topically.

Oleoresin—a natural plant product consisting of essential oil and resin extracted with alcohol, ether, or acetone. Not all the substances in the original plant are extracted, but the end result is usually more potent and more uniform.

Opiate—any derivative of opium.

Opioids—any narcotic that has opiate-like activities but is not derived from opium. They are analgesics, and suppress both the perception of and reaction to pain. Endorphins are a natural opioid produced in the body.

Osteoarthritis—noninflammatory arthritis, often called degenerative arthritis. It is manifested by destruction of joint cartilage with hypertrophy of bony margins and spur formation (osteophyte). Pain and stiffness are common complaints. It is the usual arthritis of aging, but may also be induced by trauma. Affects about sixteen million Americans.

Osteoporosis—a condition that affects about twenty-four million Americans in which bones suffer heavy losses of calcium and become brittle and easily fractured. Occurs more commonly in thin, fair, postmenopausal women. It is best diagnosed by dual photon X-ray bone densinometry. Various medications are now available for effective treatment.

Oxalate—a chemical absorbed from foods and produced in the Krebs cycle during energy production. It is excreted in the urine, and is known as a topical irritant that can cause tissue burning. Foods of plant origin, such as fruits and vegetables, are high in oxalates.

Padauk—a South American plant used in making expensive cosmetics. Blocks guaifenesin.

Palpitation—awareness of heartbeat, including irregular, forceful, or rapid beating.

Pamelor® (nortriptyline HCl)—a tricyclic antidepressant used to help with sleep problems. Can cause reverse effects and stimulate some patients.

Parathyroid glands—small glands located behind the thyroid gland that secrete parathyroid hormone, a major regulator of calcium and phosphate metabolism.

Paresthesia—altered sensation of the skin, e.g., numbness, tingling, crawling, touch, burning, coldness, etc.

Paxil® (paroxetine HCl)—a serotonin and norepinephrine reuptake inhibitor; helps cut the sensation of pain and can help with sleep.

Pentosan polysulfate (Elmiron®)—used to treat interstitial cystitis. Side effects include nausea, headaches, and diarrhea.

Percodan® (oxycodone and aspirin), Percocet® (oxycodone and acetaminophen)—strong sedative pain medications with serious potential for drug dependence and abuse. Side effects are fatigue, dizziness, sedation, and nausea.

pH—measurement of the acidity or alkalinity of a solution on a scale from 0 to 14, with 14 being the strongest alkaline reading. Body fluids are normally very near 7.4 (close to neutrality).

Phenyl salicylate—one of a combination of compounds used to treat pain and discomfort in the urinary tract in a medication called Urised®.

Phlegm—thick, sticky, stringy mucus secreted by the mucous membrane of the respiratory tract, as during a cold or respiratory infection.

Phosphates—salts containing a combination of phosphorus and another element. They are an essential part of the diet, in cereals, dairy products, eggs, and meat. Eighty-five percent of the body's phosphate is combined with calcium to form bone, and the remainder is in other body tissues. A phosphate compound provides energy for the chemical reactions in cells. Kidneys control the level of phosphates in the body, often through the process of reabsorption.

Polyethylene glycol (PEG)—a chemical used in antiperspirants, cosmetic creams, lipsticks, and fragrances. It is a petroleum byproduct and will not block guaifenesin.

Polymyalgia rheumatica—a disease marked by pain and stiffness in the muscles of the hips, thighs, shoulders, and neck, and sometimes chewing muscles (masseters). It usually occurs over the age of fifty, and affects twice as many women as men. Diagnosis is confirmed by a blood test (a sedimentation rate). It is treated with corticosteroid drugs. It may be associated with temporal arteritis, and, if untreated, can lead to blindness or stroke.

Polysaccharides—a carbohydrate consisting of a long chain of molecules. Starch and cellulose are polysaccharides.

Potaba (aminobenzoate potassium)—one of the B vitamin complex sometimes recommended for myofascial pain. Cannot be taken with sulfa drugs.

Prednisone—a synthetic glucocorticoid derived from cortisone, administered orally as an anti-inflammatory and immunosuppressant in a wide variety of disorders. It has many severe side effects and should be used only when absolutely necessary.

Prion transfer—a transmission mechanism whereby infectious proteins could be transferred from one species to another by ingestion.

Probenecid (Benemid®)—a uricosuric agent that increases the excretion of uric acid by blocking its tubular reabsorption; used in the treatment of gout. It is the first medication we used to treat fibromyalgia.

Progesterone—a steroid hormone primarily secreted by the ovary in the second half of the menstrual cycle. Its main function is to prepare the uterus for implantation of the fertilized ovum, to maintain pregnancy, and to promote development of the mammary glands. Synthetic and natural progesterones are used in conjunction with estrogens in female hormone replacement therapy to reduce the risk of uterine cancer. Adverse effects are: weight gain, edema, appetite loss, headaches, dizziness, breast tenderness, and ovarian cysts.

Prolactin (PRL)—one of the hormones secreted by the pituitary gland that stimulates and sustains lactation. A large number of other effects have been described, including essential roles in maintaining immune system functions and ovulation.

Propoxyphene—the active narcotic ingredient in Darvon® and Darvocet®—related to methadone. Dizziness, sedation, and nausea are the primary side effects. Is considered potentially addictive.

Propulsid® (cisapride)—a drug used to treat heartburn due to gastroesophageal reflux. It interacts with other medications, and should be used with care. The primary side effect is headache, but it can also cause diarrhea, gas, and abdominal pain.

Prosed®—a phenyl salicylate compound used to treat urinary tract pain. Will block guaifenesin.

ProSom® (estazolam tablets)—a sedative used for short-term treatment of insomnia. Side effects include headaches, malaise, and somnolence (in almost half of patients).

Prostaglandins—a group of hormone-like substances that mediate a wide range of physiological functions. Each has different effects such as causing uterine or bronchial muscle contractions or release of fluid. Others are mediators of inflammation.

Prostatitis—inflammation of the prostate usually seen in men between the ages of thirty and fifty. Often caused by a bacterial infection.

Prostatodynia—pain in the prostate.

Proximal renal tubules—very active area of the kidney involved in absorption and excretion of electrolytes and other metabolites.

Prozac® (fluoxetine HCl)—a specific serotonin reuptake inhibitor; antidepressant used for depression and fatigue. May cause insomnia and loss of appetite.

Pseudoephedrine—a decongestant drug used to relieve nasal congestion. It is also the active ingredient in over-the-counter appetite suppressants. Side effects include anxiety, nausea, elevated blood pressure, headaches, and palpitations. The natural form, the herb ephedra, is used as a stimulant. Ephedra will block guaifenesin, pseudoephedrine will not.

Psoriasis—a chronic skin disease characterized by red scaly, disfiguring patches.

Psychosomatic—an illness perceived to be due to body abnormalities that is actually caused or influenced by the mind.

Pycnogenol—a bioflavonoid extracted from pine bark, grapeseed, or fruits. It is also used to treat inflammation and the pain of arthritis. Will block guaifenesin.

Pyridium® (phenazopyridine HCl)—a urinary tract analgesic that is available in both prescription and over-the-counter strengths.

Quercetin—a substance found in elder flowers, blue-green algae, and quercitron bark. Used as a yellow dye and in vitamins as a bioflavonoid. The active ingredient, isoquercitin, has been found to block allergic reactions, and inhibit inflammation. Will block guaifenesin.

Questran Light® (cholestyramine)—a cholesterol-lowering agent. The primary side effects are constipation, bloating, and abdominal pain and gas.

Quillaja extract (soap bark, quillay bark, panama bark, china bark)—extract from the bark of a South American tree. Used to flavor foods such as root beer and ice cream, and as in skin products as a detergent. Blocks guaifenesin.

Raynaud's phenomenon—sensitivity of the hands and fingers to cold, with blanching, numbness, and/or pain in the fingers.

Reabsorption—the process of absorbing again substances (glucose, proteins, phosphates, etc.) already secreted into the renal tubules, and their return to the circulating blood.

Receptor—a specific area on the surface or nucleus of a cell with a characteristic structure. It recognizes and binds a molecule of appropriate size, shape, and charge. Receptors are activated by chemicals, hormones, or drugs. Many drugs are designed to occupy receptors and thus block an action.

Relafen® (nabumetone)—a nonsteroidal anti-inflammatory drug. It is absorbed in the intestine and can be used on those patients who experience gastric upset with other drugs in this class. May cause elevated liver enzymes and gastric bleeding.

Restless leg syndrome—burning, prickling, or uncomfortable sensations in the muscles of the legs which tend to occur at night in bed, or when sitting in a prolonged, dependent-leg position, such as on an airplane or in a theater. Restless leg syndrome is thought to affect fifteen percent of the population, and is more common in women than in men.

Reversal—movement in the opposite direction (backwards).

Rheumatism—a term for any disorder that can cause musculoskeletal pain or stiffness.

Rheumatoid arthritis—a chronic disease marked by stiffness and joint inflammation. Damage may lead to a loss of mobility and deformity. It affects two to three times more women than men—about 2.1 million Americans.

Robinul® (glycopyrrolate)—an anticholinergic drug used to treat ulcers. It is uricosuric. Side effects include fatigue, headaches, and weakness. We have used it to treat fibromyalgia.

Rolfing—a very rough form of massage therapy.

Salicin—a chemical derived from the bark of several species of willow and poplar trees. Aspirin and other salicylates are derived from salicin, or made synthetically. Blocks guaifenesin.

Salicylates—salts of salicylic acid (amyl, phenyl, benzyl, menthyl, glyceryl, diproplene glycol esters). Occur naturally in all plants. Used as sunburn preventatives, analgesics.

Salicylic acid (Methyl salicylate)—occurs naturally in wintergreen, sweet birch, and other plants. It can be absorbed through the skin. It is used as an exfolient, preservative, fungicide, and antiseptic agent. Blocks guaifenesin.

Sarcoplasm—the nonfibrillar cytoplasm of a muscle fiber.

Seborrhea—excessive secretion of sebum causing an increased oiliness of the face and scalp.

Seborrheic dermatitis—a red scaly rash that develops on the face, scalp, chest, and back. On the scalp it is the most common cause of dandruff. The exact cause of the rash is unknown.

Sedative—a drug having a soothing, calming, or tranquilizing effect. Sedatives include sleeping drugs, antianxiety drugs, antipsychotic drugs, and antidepressant drugs.

Serotonin—a neurotransmitter thought to play a part in temperature regulation, mood, and sleep. Found in many tissues of the body including the brain, but especially blood platelets. It inhibits secretions in the digestive tract, stimulates smooth muscle, and affects appetite.

Serotonin reuptake inhibitors—a group of antidepressant medications that slow the withdrawal of serotonin from activated brain sites. This prolongs the effects of serotonin.

Serum—the clear portion of the blood separated from its solid elements.

Shea butter—natural fat from the fruit of the karite tree. Used in soap and candles. Will not block guaifenesin.

Sigmoid colon—the lower portion of the colon.

Sigmoidoscopy—an examination of the lower portion of the colon, using a fiber-optic instrument known as a sigmoidoscope.

Sinequan® (doxepin HCl)—a tricyclic antidepressant and antihistamine which causes sedation. It can also be used to control muscle twitching. Side effects include fatigue and dizziness.

Sodium cocyl isethionate—the sodium salt of the coconut fatty acid esther of isethionate acid.

Sodium salicylate—a nonsteroidal anti-inflammatory drug.

Soma® (carisoprodol)—a central nervous system depressant that causes muscles to relax, and can also help with the sensory overload symptoms of fibromyalgia. It can cause drowsiness and raise the seizure threshold.

Soma Compound®—same as above, but contains aspirin and cannot be used with guaifenesin.

Sorbitol—a white crystalline alcohol, found in various berries and fruits or made synthetically, used as a flavoring agent, a sugar substitute for people with diabetes, and a moisturizer in cosmetics and other products.

Stearic acid—occurs naturally in butter acids, tallow, bark, and other animal fats and oils. A large percentage of cosmetic creams contain stearic acid, which is what gives creams their pearly appearance.

Stearyl alcohol (stenol)—a mixture of solid alcohols prepared from sperm whale oil. Will not block guaifenesin.

Steroids—compounds of hormonal origin such as cortisone; used to treat inflammation caused by allergies.

Substance P—present in nerve cells throughout the body and in certain endocrine cells in the gut; it increases the contractions of gastrointestinal smooth muscle and causes vasodilation. It is a sensory neurotransmitter mediating touch and temperature, and alerts the body to pain.

Sulfinpyrazone (Anturane®)—a medicine used in the treatment of gout. It is uricosuric which means that it causes the kidneys to excrete more uric acid. It was the second medication we used to treat fibromyalgia.

Sumatriptan (Imitrex®)—selected serotonin antagonist used in the treatment of migraine headaches. Can be administered by injection, pill, or nasal spray. Common side effects are nausea and tightness in the chest.

Syncope—the medical term for fainting.

Syndrome—a group of symptoms and signs that occur together and constitute a particular disorder.

Systemic—affecting the entire body, rather than just a part of it.

Tagamet® (cimetidine)—a histamine$_2$ blocker (H$_2$ blocker) used to decrease stomach acidity. Prescribed also for gastroesophageal reflux. Can also help with sleep.

Tartar—a hard, yellowish deposit on the teeth, consisting of organic secretions and food particles deposited with various salts, such as calcium and phosphate.

T cells—a type of white blood cell that plays a major role in the body's immune system.

Temporomandibular joint syndrome (TMJ)—pain and other symptoms of the head, jaw, neck, and face stemming from the muscles and ligaments surrounding the joint where the lower jaw attaches to the head at the temporal bone.

Tender points—the official definition of FMS states that patients must have tenderness in eleven out of eighteen predetermined sites (and these must be in all four quadrants of the body). Tender points hurt intensely when they are pressed on.

Tendon—a band of strong nonelastic fibrous tissue that is cord-like. It is the stretched end of a muscle where it attaches to bone, cartilage or skin.

Thyroid—an endocrine gland. It is the body's metabolic thermostat and controls temperature, energy use, and in children, the growth rate. It controls the rate at which organs function; it affects the operation of all body processes and organs.

Titrate—to determine the proper amount of medication needed for therapeutic action by gradually and systematically raising the dosage until the desired effect has occurred.

Topical—a substance applied to any body surface. Also refers to substances applied inside the ear canal, the surface of the eye, or inserted vaginally or rectally such as suppositories.

Tramadol (Ultram®)—a medication for moderate to severe pain. It is one of a new class of drugs known as CABAs (centrally acting binary agents). It has a low abuse potential compared to narcotic analgesics. Side effects include nausea and the lowering of the seizure threshold.

Transdermal—administration of a drug applied to the skin in ointment or patch form; the drug passes through the skin into the bloodstream.

Traumatic arthritis—joint pain caused by damage from an accident.

Tremor—trembling or quivering of muscles, usually noted in the hands or head.

TRH—a hormone of the brain that stimulates the release of TSH. It is also a neurotransmitter.

Tricyclic antidepressant drugs—the most widely used class of antidepressants, named for their three-ring molecular structure.

Trigger points—painful areas of the body that can induce spasm in adjacent muscles or radiate pain to other regions that are served by the same nerves.

Triglyceride—one of three "blood fats" that are known as lipids. It is the principal constituent of body fat. It is manufactured in the liver largely from sugar and starches, and deposited in fat cells for energy storage.

Tryptophan—an amino acid first isolated from milk in 1901. Dietary tryptophan is the precursor to serotonin, an important neurotransmitter, as well as melatonin. Over-the-counter tryptophan was withdrawn from the market in 1990 because of more than a thousand cases of eosinophilia myalgia syndrome. The problem was found to be a contaminant in the tablet and not with the amino acid itself.

TSH—a hormone secreted by the pituitary gland in response to TRH. It promotes growth of the thyroid gland and secretion of thyroid hormone.

Tuckability—a word coined for this book referring to the ability of the body to store accumulated calcium and phosphate.

Ultram® (tramadol HCl)—one of a new class of pain medications, it is a CABA (centrally acting binary agent). It has a low abuse potential when compared to codeine. Side effects include nausea and the lowering of the seizure threshold.

Ultrasound—high-frequency sound waves used to study solid structures within the body such as the liver, heart, pancreas, etc. The waves are converted to images by a transducer for imaging and interpretation. These waves cannot pass through bones or make images of gas.

Unised®—a combination of analgesics including phenyl salicylate; used to treat pain and discomfort in the urinary tract. Will block guaifenesin.

Urethritis—inflammation of the urethra, usually due to an infection. It causes a burning sensation when passing urine (dysuria). There may be traces of blood in the urine.

Uric acid—a product from the breakdown of nucleic acids in body cells, also produced in the digestion of some foods, the end product of purine catabolism. Gout is caused by the deposition of sodium urate crystals in the joints. Uric acid is also known as a powerful antioxidant.

Uricosuric—a drug that causes the kidneys to increase the excretion of uric acid.

Vaginosis—a disease of the vagina that may have positive cultures for gardnerella or mobiluncus characterized by a gray vaginal discharge.

Vicodin® (hydrocodone bitartrate)—a codeine derivative in combination with acetaminophen (Tylenol) that is used for severe pain. It is a habit-forming and commonly abused drug. Side effects include lightheadedness, dizziness, sedation, constipation, nausea, and vomiting.

Voltaren® (diclofenac sodium)—a nonsteroidal anti-inflammatory drug with analgesic and antipyretic properties used to treat muscle pain and menstrual cramps.

Vulva—the external female genitalia including the clitoris and the labia.

Vulvar pain (vulvodynia)—excruciating pain, burning, and/or itching in the vulvar area. Patients may have difficult in walking, intercourse (dyspareunia), or even sitting. It is estimated to afflict between 150,000 and 200,000 women in the United States.

Vulvar vestibulitis syndrome—a pain syndrome characterized by pain in the area of the vestibule, or entrance to the vagina. It may cause dyspareunia, or painful sexual intercourse.

Vulvitis—inflammation of the vulva. Symptoms include redness, itching, and swelling. Blisters may form and ooze, forming a crusty surface.

Vulvodynia—a syndrome which often includes vulvitis (raw, irritated, burning vaginal lips) and vulvar pain, vaginal spasms or cramps, burning discharge, increased menstrual and uterine cramps, painful intercourse (dyspareunia), repeated bladder infections, burning urination (dysuria), pungent urine, and chronic interstitial cystitis.

Vulvovaginitis (candidal and noncandidal)—irritation and inflammation of the vulvar area and the vagina. Candidal vulvovaginitis is characterized by a cottage-cheese-like discharge and the presence of candida albicans, a yeast fungus.

X ray—a type of electromagnetic radiation that is absorbed by dense structures such as bone. Used to diagnose conditions such as osteoarthritis and bone spurs, abnormalities that are irreversible.

Yucca—an evergreen plant native to the warmer regions of North America; used in shampoos and soaps.

Zantac® (ranitidine hydrochloride)—a histamine$_2$ blocker that inhibits basal gastric acid secretion. Used to treat gastritis and stomach ulcers. The predominant side effects are headaches, nausea, constipation, and lethargy.

Resources

FIBROMYALGIA (CHAPTER 2)

Books

Copeland, Mary Ellen, and Wayne London. *The Depression Workbook.* Oakland: New Harbinger, 1992.

Starlanyl, Devin J., M.D. *The Fibromyalgia Advocate: Getting the Support You Need to Cope with Fibromyalgia.* Oakland: New Harbinger, 1998.

Starlanyl, Devin J., M.D., and Mary Ellen Copeland. *Fibromyalgia & Chronic Myofascial Pain Syndrome.* Oakland: New Harbinger, 1996.

Williamson, Miryam Erlich. *Fibromyalgia: A Comprehensive Approach.* New York: Walker & Co., 1998.

____. *The Fibromyalgia Relief Book.* New York: Walker & Co., 1998.

Multimedia

CD ROM—*Body Pain Trigger Points Program Volume One.* $39.99 (MAC and Microsoft Windows format). To order call (310) 215-9816. Based on the studies of Dr. Travell and Dr. Simons and

shows the common trigger points and the patterns of pain they produce.

Videotape—*Chronic Myofascial Pain Syndrome: A Guide to the Trigger Points.* Dr. Devin J. Starlanyl, M.D. New Harbinger Publications, 1977.

Newsgroups/Support Groups

FMS Recovery List: A private, semi-moderated support group.
Owner: Tesa Marcon. To subscribe send an e-mail to LIST-
SERVE@MAELSTROM.STJOHNS.EDU and type in the command
SUB FMS-RECOVERY RealFirstName, RealLastName in the
body of the e-mail.

(This is *not* the Guai-Support list.)

FIBROM-L or alt.med.fibromyalgia—This is the largest FM on-line
group, but is not as supportive of the Guaifenesin protocol as is
the Guai List, below. To subscribe send an e-mail to list-
serv@mitvma.mit.edu and in the body of the message type sub
FIBROM-L and your first and last name.

Web Sites

Fibromyalgia and Myofascial Pain Syndrome: by Dr. Devin J. Starlanyl, M.D.
www.sover.net/~devstar
A Fibromyalgia Web site: by Miryam Williamson
www.shaysnet.com/~wmson/

Associations

The Arthritis Foundation, National Office (404) 872-7100
1330 W. Peachtree St., Atlanta, GA 30309 www.arthritis.org

The Arthritis Foundation of Canada (416) 967-1414
National Headquarters, 250 Bloor Street East #901, Toronto, ON M4W 3P2

Association de la Fibromyosite du Quebec, 60 Rue Notre Dame, Repentigny, PQ J6A 2W1 Canada. Fibromyalgia Information in French.

Fibromialgia Fundacion Mexicana (FIBRO) (525) 528-25-95 ext 14
Alejandro Carmona, Director. Moctezuma 26, col. Jose Toriello guerra, c.p. 14050, Delegacion Tlalpan, Mex, DF e-mail: recursos@vitalmex.com.mx

GUAIFENESIN PROTOCOL (CHAPTER 3)

Guaifenesin Users' Support Group

Fibromyalgia Wellness Group (212) 832-8352, New York City.
Contact: Aileen Goldberg or e-mail at www.Gold2222@aol.com. Meets twice monthly.

On-Line: The "Guai Support Group" List
To Subscribe send an e-mail to: LISTSERV@MAELSTROM. STJOHNS.EDU and type: Sub Guai-Support (Your First name) (Your Last name) in the body of the e-mail. This is a private semi-moderated support group for anyone interested in the guaifenesin protocol and hypoglycemia. Also provides salicylate information. Members are in all stages of treatment. Founded by Tesa Marcon in October 1997. Six hundred plus members in all stages of recovery.

Guaifenesin Support Web Sites

The Guai Group: www.geocities.com/HotSprings/Spa/5252 "Official" support and information for the guaifenesin protocol. Site contains updated cosmetic lists, success stories, doctors list, etc. Appropriate for doctors and patients.

R. Paul St. Amand, M.D. and Claudia Marek's Web site: www. fibromyalgiatreatment.com Guaifenesin treatment updates, referral lists, and links to other resources.

Fibromeet by Nancy Medeiros: www.csusm.edu/public/guests/nancym/fibromt A patient-oriented Web site with a folksy look. Offers video-tapes and other information for sale.

Videotapes

R. Paul St. Amand, M.D. and Claudia Marek. Video of a speech in 1998 to a support group in San Diego. Also a tape demonstrating Dr. St. Amand's mapping technique. *Dr. St. Amand and Claudia Marek receive no compensation of any kind for the making or sales of these videotapes. In recognition of this fact, Fibromeet has agreed to donate $2.00 for every videotape purchased to THE FIBROMYALGIA TREATMENT FUND, a non-profit organization.* Fibromeet: P.O. Box 461377, Escondido, CA 92046-1377 www.csusm.edu/public/guests/nancym/fibromt.htm The Treatment of Fibromyalgia with Guaifenesin $23.20. Mapping Fibromyalgia $13.20. (Prices include shipping and handling.)

Success Stories

Sometimes it helps to hear about another person's success. Here are three good sites:

www.geocities.com/HotSprings/Spa/5252/successstories.html
www.sover.net/~devstar/relative.htm
www.csusm.edu/public/guests/nancym/fibromt.htm

Guaifenesin Sources

Bemis Drug (781) 878-0893
> Contact Bill Sells. 200 mg pills without prescription, 600 mg tablets with prescription.

College Pharmacy (800) 888-9358
> Pete Hueseman, Pharmacist. Sells 600 mg pills with prescription. Fax (719) 262-0036. Colorado Springs, CO.

Health Products Express, Inc. (800) 846-5525
> Sells 200 mg guaifenesin without a prescription. Located in Massachusetts. www.healthpx.com

Hyrex Pharmaceuticals (800) 238-5282
> Sells Hytuss (guaifenesin) 200 mg over the counter. Located in Memphis, TN.

Marina del Rey Pharmacy (310) 823-5311
> Jim Zelenay, Pharmacist. 4558 So. Admiralty Way, Marina del Rey, CA 90292. Fax (310) 577-7562. Will ship guaifenesin worldwide to those with a prescription. Also has information on salicylate-free skin care and samples in pharmacy.

Medi-Mail (800) 422-6579
> Phone number for physicians to call in prescriptions: (800) 648-6834, Las Vegas, NV.

Unicare Pharmacy (800) 438-2014
> 600 mg tablets with a prescription. Located in Omaha, NE.

Canada: (*Guaifenesin in Canada does not require a prescription but it also does not come in tablet form.*) You can mail your prescription to the U.S. or buy the powder and fill your own capsules. Fludan Fine Chemicals Inc. (613) 678-5837 sells both powder and empty capsules. The pharmacist can help you figure out how much to put in them. They ship all over Canada and also to the U.S. www.hawk.igs.net/~franika. Powder is also available from

Valtrec, which has branches in Vancouver, Montreal, and Toronto.

SALICYLATES (CHAPTER 4)

Salicylate-Free Skin Care

Andrea Rose Salicylate-Free Skin Care and lipsticks (888) 712-ROSE. www.andrearose.com

Compounding Pharmacies (*to assist with salicylate-free topicals, etc.*)

Compounding Pharmacy of Beverly Hills (888) 799-0212
  9629 W. Olympic Blvd., Beverly Hills, CA 90212

International Academy of Compounding Pharmacists
(800) 927-4227

Women's International Pharmacy
(800) 279-5708 (800) 279-8011 fax

This is a nonprofit organization representing pharmacists who compound custom medications to meet unique patient needs. The number is for referrals to pharmacists.

COSMETIC COMPANY CUSTOMER SERVICE PHONE NUMBERS/WEB SITES

Adrien Arpel (212) 333-7700
www.adrienarpel.com

Alexandra de Markoff
(800) 4-REVLON

Almay (800) 4-REVLON

Alpha Hydroxy/Neoteric
(800) 55-ALPHA
www.alpha-hydrox.com

Avon (800) 367-2866
www.avon.com

Basis (800) 926-4832

BeautiControl (800) 624-4573
www.beauti.com/index.html

Bobbi Brown (212) 980-7040
www.bobbibrowncosmetics.com

The Body Shop (800) 541-2535
www.the-body-shop.com

Borghese (212) 572-3100

Cetaphil
www.cetaphil.com

Chanel (212) 688-5055

Charles of the Ritz (800) 4-REVLON

Christian Dior (212) 759-1840

Clarins (212) 980-1800

Clearasil www.clearasil.com

Clinique (212) 572-3800
www.clinique.com

Coty (212) 850-2300

Cover Girl (800) 426-8374
www.covergirl.com

DermaBlend (905) 660-0622
www.sheen.com/derma/dblend.html

Donna Karan (800) 647-7474

Dove (800) 451-6679

Elizabeth Arden (212) 261-1000

Erno Laszlo (415) 341-0925

Estée Lauder (212) 756-4801

Eucerin (800) 227-4703

Galderma (800) 582-8225
www.galderma.com/products/usa

Guerlain (212) 751-1870
www.guerlain.com

Iman (212) 750-6776
www.sheen.com/iman/iman.htm

Jafra (800) 551-2345

Jergens (800) 222-3553

Johnson & Johnson (800) 526-3967

La Prairie (800) 821-5718
www.laprairie.com

Lancome (800) 526-2663
www.lancome.com

L'Oreal (800) 322-2036
www.lorealcosmetics.com

Lubriderm (800) 223-0182
www.skinhelp.com

M.A.C. (800) 387-6707

Mary Kay (800) 627-9529
www.marykay.com

Max Factor (800) 862-4222

Maybelline (901) 320-4778

M.D. Formulations (800) 55-FORTE

Merle Norman (800) 348-8889

Monteil of Paris (212) 593-7400

Murad (800) 242-1103

NeoStrata (800) 628-9904
www.neostrata.com/index/html

Neutrogena (800) 421-6857
www.neutrogena.com

Nivea (800) 233-2340
www.nivea.com

Oil of Olay (800) 285-5170

Physicians Formula (800) 227-0333
www.physiciansformula.com

Pond's (800) 243-5804

Prescriptives (212) 756-4801

Purpose (800) 526-3967

Revlon (800) 4-REVLON
www.revlon.com

Shiseido (212) 805-2300

Trish McEvoy (212) 758-7790

Ultima II (800) 4-REVLON

Urban Decay
www.urbandecay.com

Vaseline Intensive Care (800) 743-8640

Victoria Jackson (800) V-MAKEUP
www.vmakeup.com

Yves St. Laurent (212) 621-7300

Books

Begoun, Paula. *Don't Go to the Cosmetic Counter without Me, 4th Edition.* Seattle, WA: Beginning Press, 1994.

PDR for Herbal Medicines. Montvale, NJ: Medical Economics, 1998.

Winter, Ruth, M.S. *The Concise Dictionary of Cosmetic Ingredients, 4th Edition.* New York: Crown, 1994.

Web Sites

American Academy of Dermatology: www.AAD.org

Dermatology On-line Journal:
http://www.matrix.ucdavis.edu/DOJdesk/desk.html

Food and Drug Administration: www.FDA.gov

Paula Begoun: www.cosmeticscop.com

Ruth Winter, M.S.: www.brain.body.com
Update on cosmetic ingredients, free newsletter.

Other Information

Cosmetic Ingredient Review Board (202) 331-0651
1101 17th Street NW suite 310, Washington, DC 20036-4702

HYPOGLYCEMIA (CHAPTER 5)

Associations

Hypoglycemia Association (202) 544-4044
P.O. Box 165, Ashton, MD 20861-4044
Meetings and materials on hypoglycemia for physicians and patients.

National Hypoglycemia Association (201) 670-1189
P.O. Box 120, Ridgewood, NJ 07451
Information, support services, and referrals to hypoglycemics, their families, and the general public.

Web Sites

Hypoglycemia Support Foundation, Inc.: www.hypoglycemia.org

Low-carbohydrate food, recipes: www.lowcarb.com

The Atkins Diet Web site: www.atkins.com

Low-Carbohydrate Resource Center: www.thinner.com

Many good recipes: www.elainecase.com/eclowcarb

Recipes, foods and ingredients: www.blackdirt.net/lowcarb

Glycemic Index of Foods: www.medosa.com/gi.html—Web's most complete resource.

Low-Carbohydrate Products

Atkins' Diet Products—www.atkins.com

Da Vinci Sugar-free Syrups (800) 640-6779—18 flavors
www.greatfood.com

Diet Depot, Inc. (877) 260-8361 toll free or www.dietdepot.com

D'lites of Shadowood (888) 937-5262 or www.lowcarb.com

La Tortilla Factory (800) 446-1516
Low Carb Tortillas. Only 3 grams of carb in their fat-free
whole-wheat, oat-fiber tortillas.

Phyl's Nutritional Corner Store (302) 738-4008 or www.magpage.
com/~paw

Splenda™ (sucralose) Low-Carbohydrate Sweetener—FDA approved but not yet available in the U.S. Made from sugar, modified so it can't be absorbed by the body. You should buy the
boxed sucralose, not the small packets that contain dextrose. It
is legal to have it sent to you from Canada. (Manufacturer is:
McNeil Specialty Company (908) 524-6336.) Can be ordered
from Global Drugs: www.globaldrugs.com Phone: (403) 246-
1227. Address: 6448 Old Banff Coach Road S.W., Calgary, AB,
T3H Canada 2H4

Stasero International, Inc. (206) 328-0690
Stasero Premium Quality Italian Style Syrup, 2001 S. Plum St.,
Seattle, WA 98144. Sugar Free (0 Carbs)—add to drinks, cof-
fee, and use in cooking.

Stevia: Herb used as a low-carbohydrate sweetener. Has a bitter
after-taste. You can use the leaves directly off the plant. Supposedly more than thirty times sweeter than sugar. Available at most
nurseries or at health-food stores. You can mail-order it from
Richter's (905) 640-6677. (Small amounts will not block guaifenesin.)

Sugar-Free Market Place: www.sugarfreemarket.com

Sugar-Free Marketplace: www.icaneat.net/sugarfree/

Low-Carbohydrate On-line Groups:

Low-carb newsgroup: www.listporc@eskimo.com Low Carb Group: To subscribe send a message to www.lowcarb-list-request@ eskimo.com and in the subject title ask to subscribe.

Low-Carb Support Group: www.alt.support.diet.low-carb Send e-mail to LISTSERV@MAELSTROM.STJOHNS.EDU and in the body of the message type SUB LOWCARB-LIST YourFirstName, YourLastName

Books

(All low-carbohydrate diets are not the same. Be sure to check all recipes to make sure they are compatible with our diet.)

Atkins, Robert C. *Dr. Atkins' New Diet Revolution.* New York: M. Evans & Co., 1992.

Everyday Low Carb Cookery: Low Carbohydrate Recipes for the 90s and Beyond by Alex Haas. Send $19.95 plus shipping and handling ($5.00 U.S., $7.00 Canada) to Alex Haas, P.O. Box 7802, Talleyville, DE 19803-7802.

Sugarfree New Orleans—A Cookbook based on the Glycemic Index by Deanie Comeaux Bahan. AFM Publishing, 1998. www.toutsuite.com

For diabetic patients:

Bernstein, Richard K. *Dr. Bernstein's Diabetes Solution.* New York: Little Brown and Co., 1997. www.diabetes-normalsugars.com

McCullough, Fran. *The Low-Carb Cookbook*. New York: Hyperion, 1997.
www.blackdirt.net/lowcarb

Book No Longer in Print

Grad, Marcia. *A Taste for Life. Recipes for a High-Protein Diet*. (Introduction by R. Paul St. Amand, M.D.). New York: Charles Scribner's Sons, 1975.

RESOURCES FOR PART II

Interstitial Cystitis/Irritable Bladder

The IC Network (707) 538-9442
   Jill Osborne, Founder, 4773 Sonoma Hwy., #125, Santa Rosa, CA 95409 www.sonic.net/jill/icnet/welcome/html

Interstitial Cystitis Association (212) 979-6057
   P.O. Box 1553, Madison Square Station, New York, NY 10159 www.ichelp.com

Interstitial Cystitis Association (310) 967-5034
   120 S. Spaulding Drive #210, Beverly Hills, CA 90212

Vulvar Pain/Vulvodynia

National Vulvodynia Association (301) 299-0775

   Phyllis Mate, Executive Director, P.O. Box 4491, Silver Spring, MD 20914-4491

   www.nva.org

The Vulvar Pain Foundation (336) 226-0704
    Director, P.O. Drawer 177, Graham, NC 27253 www.
    vulvarpainfoundation.org

For Treatment

Scripps Pain Center Vulvar Pain Program (619) 626-4337
    Scripps Clinic and Research Foundation, 10666 N. Torrey
    Pines Rd., La Jolla, CA 92037

John J. Williems, M.D. (619) 554-8690
    Scripps Clinic and Research Foundation, 10666 N. Torrey
    Pines Rd., La Jolla, CA 92037

Book

The Low Oxalate Cookbook (The VP Foundation). Edited by Meg
    Stolzfus and Joanne J. Yount. The Vulvar Pain Foundation,
    1997. $30.00 including postage and handling.
    www.vulvarpainfoundation.org

Gastrointestinal Disorders

International Foundation for Functional Gastrointestinal Disorders
(888) 964-2001
P.O. Box 17864, Milwaukee, WI 53217
www.execpc.com//iffgd
Support and educational services, referral listings, and facilitates support groups.

Intestinal Disease Foundation, Inc. (412) 261-5888
1323 Forbes Ave #200, Pittsburgh, PA 15219
Support groups, telephone support network.

National Digestive Diseases Information Clearinghouse
(301) 654-3810
2 Information Way, Bethesda, MD 20892-3570
e-mail:nddic@aerie.com

Web Sites

For bowel disorders: www.qurlyjoe.bu.edu/cduchome.html

The IBS page: www.panix.com/~ibs

IBS Self Help Group: www.ibsgroup.org

Other Associations

National Headache Foundation (800) 843-2256
5252 North Western Ave., Chicago, IL 60625
Relaxation tapes, information on headaches.

Restless Leg Syndrome
4410 19th Street NW #201, Rochester, MN 55901
www.rls.org

The TMJ Association (414) 259-8112
P.O. Box 26770, Milwaukee, WI 53226
www.tmj.org

RESOURCES FOR PART III (THE ROAD BACK)

Physical Therapy

Acupressure Institute (510) 854-1059
1533 Shattuck Avenue, Berkeley, CA 94709

Alexander Technique (217) 367-6956
P.O. Box 517, Urbana, IL 61801
www.alexandertechnique.com

American Academy of Physical Medicine and Rehabilitation
(312) 464-9700
One IBM Plaza #2500, Chicago, IL 60611-3065

American Chiropractic Association (703) 276-8800
1701 Clarendon Bl, Arlington, VA 22209

American Massage Therapy Association (847) 864-0123
802 Davis Street #100, Evanston, IL 60201-4444
www.lightlink.com

American Physical Therapy Association (703) 684-2782
111 N. Fairfax St., Alexandria, VA 22314

Feldenkrais Guild (800) 775-2118
P.O. Box 489, Albany, OR 97321-0143
www.feldenkrais.com

Treatment

Pauline Sugine (310) 281-6106
10780 Santa Monica Blvd. #450
Los Angeles, CA 90026
Will refer to other practitioners.

Relaxation

Deer Mountain T'ai Chi Health Academy
P.O. Box 19835, Asheville, NC 28815
Relaxation and meditation tapes.

Serenity (800) 869-1684
180 W. 25th Street, Upland, CA 91786
Relaxation tapes.

Exercise: Video Tapes

Gentle Fitness (800) 566-7780
732 Lake Shore Drive, Rhinelander, WI 54501
Award-winning video tape comes with helpful 20-page book. By
Catherine MacRae. Blends Yoga, T'ai Chi and Feldenkrais movement awareness. $28.70 including postage. www.gentlefitness.com

Improving Muscle Tone and Strength: A Fibromyalgia Fitness Tape by Dr. Sharon Clark. Also: Dr. Sharon Clark's Stretching Video. Oregon FM Foundation, 1221 Yamhill, suite 303, Portland, OR 97205. $25.00 each, including shipping. (Also available in European format.)

Stretching, Inc. (800) 315-1995
Bob and Jean Anderson, P.O. Box 767, Palmer Lake, CO 80222-9050

Miscellaneous Help

How to Run A Support Group by Bev. Spencer, National Foundation for FM, P.O. Box 3429, San Diego, CA 91263-1429

National Self-Help Clearing House (212) 354-8525
25 W. 43rd Street, room 620, New York, NY 10036

The United States Department of Justice Americans with Disabilities Act (ADA)
Home Page: www.usdoj.gov/crt/ada/adahom1.htm

U.S. Equal Employment Opportunity Commission Publication and Information Center (800) 669-3362
P.O. Box 12549, Cincinnati, OH 45212-0549

For significant others

Well Spouse Foundation (800) 838-0879
601 Lexington Ave., suite 813, New York, NY 10022
Bi-monthly newsletter & other support.

Well Spouse Foundation (619) 673-9043
P.O. Box 28876, San Diego, CA 92198
Support groups, newsletter.

Doctors List

This is a partial list of doctors who use guaifenesin and have worked with Dr. St. Amand. An updated list is available on www.fibromyalgia-treatment.com *or by sending a SASE to R. Paul St. Amand, M.D. 4560 Admiralty Way, suite 355, Marina del Rey, CA 90292*

Dr. R. Paul St. Amand, M.D. (310) 577-7510
4560 Admiralty Way, suite 355, Marina del Rey, CA 90292

Deb Brandt, N.P. (605) 342-3280
Rapid City Medical Center, 2820 Mt. Rushmore Rd., Rapid City, SD 57701

Dr. Matt Brunson, M.D. (205) 664-8292
1006 1st Street N, Alabaster, AL 35007

Dr. John A. Gatell, M.D. (770) 804-6440
Atlanta Pain Relief Center, 400 Perimeter Terrace Center
Atlanta, GA 30346 infoedrgatell.com

Dr. Kendall J. Gerdes, M.D. (303) 977-8837
#2 Steele Street #200, Denver, CO 80206

John G. Hipps, M.D. (814) 834-2605
RRI North Creek, Emporium, PA 15834

Dr. Steven Levy, D.O. (713) 451-4100
1140 Westmont #300, Houston, TX 77015

Dr. Cynthia Palmisano, M.D. (847) 985-9106
1080 Nerge Road, Elk Grove, IL 60007

Dr. Bruce Solitar, M.D. (212) 889-7217
333 E. 34th St. #1C, New York, NY 10016

Dr. Walter Ward, M.D. (336) 760-0240
1411-B Plaza West, Winston-Salem, NC 27103

Index

Smythe, Hugh, 8, 20, 200
Social Security, 11, 144, 261–62
sodium, 51, 68, 83, 88
Solitar, Bruce M., xii
Solomons, Clive, 178
Soma (carisoprodol), 67, 89, 195, 244, 258
somnolence, 257–58
spearmint, 85, 94
spices, 120, 138–39
starches, 83, 100–101, 103, 111, 304–5
  in FMS, 130, 192
  in hypoglycemia, 115–17, 149–50
  in IBS, 191–92
Starlanyl, Devin J., 39, 199, 210, 275, 277–78
Stolle, Mary Ellen, 95
stress, 306, 315
  reduction of, 266–74, 281–82
strict low-carbohydrate diet, 140
Strobel, E. S., 312–13
sugars, 100–101, 304–5
  in fibroglycemia, 132, 137–38, 140–42
  in FMS, 4, 113, 130, 132, 134–35, 192
  in hypoglycemia, 96–97, 102–7, 109, 11118, 124, 146, 149–50, 267, 270
  in IBS, 191–92, 197
sulfinpyrazone (Anturane), 41, 47–49
sumatriptan, 230–31
support groups, 146, 151, 157, 179
  in coping with FMS, 275–76
sweating, 113
  in hypoglycemia, 97, 104, 106–7, 109, 111, 149
Sydenham, Thomas, 41–43

tartar, 39–40, 45–47, 77, 307
tender points, *see* lumps and bumps
thyroid, 20, 37, 146, 253
tingling, *see* numbness and tingling
toothpastes, 88
topical preparations, 87, 89–90
toxins, 67, 92

tramadol (Ultram), 245, 258
tranquilizers, 257–58, 267
tremors, 104, 106–7, 111, 149
tricyclic medications, 242–43, 249–51
triglycerides, 83, 102–3
Tylenol, 67, 220, 230–31, 237, 246, 249, 254–55

Ultram (tramadol), 245, 258
ultrasound, 184–85, 245
University Hospital in London, 7
University of California at Los Angeles (UCLA), 100
urates, 306–7
urethra, 167–68
uric acid:
  in FMS, 54–55
  in gout, 41–47, 49, 55
  guaifenesin in lowering levels of, 49–50
uricosuric medications, 41, 47, 75, 135, 305–8
urination:
  in bladder infections and irritations, 168–70, 172–74
  in FMS, 113
  in pediatric fibromyalgia, 232
  in vaginal problems, 178

vaginal problems, 167–68, 172–84
vegetables:
  in diets for fibroglycemia, 137–39
  in diets for hypoglycemia, 119, 122
vitamins, 5, 78, 94, 155, 253–54
  C, 95, 173
vulvar pain, 203
  in FMS, 6–7, 20–21, 25, 28, 46, 167, 174–83
  in pediatric fibromyalgia, 235
Vulvar Pain Foundation, 95, 177–83
vulvar vestibulitis syndrome (VVS), 174–76
vulvodynia, 197
  in FMS, 25, 113, 172–77, 179–83

R. PAUL ST. AMAND, M.D., is a graduate of Tufts University School of Medicine. He has been on the teaching staff at the Los Angeles Harbor/UCLA Hospital, Department of Endocrinology for over forty-three years. He is currently an assistant clinical professor at the UCLA School of Medicine. Dr. St. Amand discovered guaifenesin's use as a treatment for fibromyalgia, and his work is cited wherever the substance is mentioned.

CLAUDIA CRAIG MAREK, M.A., is a medical assistant tutored, trained, and taught on the job by Dr. St. Amand. She has co-written medical papers with Dr. St. Amand and has counseled fibromyalgia patients for more than ten years.